rr092

1001 MULTIPL
QUESTIONS AN
IN SURC

CU00686474

1001 Multiple Choice Questions and Answers in Surgery

A companion to surgical study
based on
Bailey & Love's Short Practice of Surgery
Edited by C.V. Mann, R.C.G. Russell and N.S. Williams

Fourth edition

BY

A.J. HARDING RAINS, CBE, MS, FRCS

Former editor, *Bailey & Love's Short Practice of Surgery*
13th–20th editions
Former examiner Primary FRCS, MRCS and FRCS England,
for the Professional and Linguistics Assessment Board,
General Medical Council and the Universities of
London, Belfast, Birmingham and Newcastle;
Professor of Surgery, University of London at
Charing Cross Hospital; Dean, British Postgraduate Medical
Federation; Vice-President and Member of Council,
Royal College of Surgeons of England

CHAPMAN & HALL MEDICAL

London · Weinheim · New York · Tokyo · Melbourne · Madras

Published by Chapman & Hall, 2–6 Boundary Row, London SE1 8HN, UK

Chapman & Hall, 2–6 Boundary Row, London SE1 8HN, UK

Chapman & Hall GmbH, Pappelallee 3, 69469 Weinheim, Germany

Chapman & Hall USA, 115 Fifth Avenue, New York, NY 10003, USA

Chapman & Hall Japan, ITP-Japan, Kyowa Building, 3F, 2-2-1 Hirakawacho, Chiyoda-ku, Tokyo 102, Japan

Chapman & Hall Australia, 102 Dodds Street, South Melbourne, Victoria 3205, Australia

Chapman & Hall India, R. Seshadri, 32 Second Main Road, CIT East, Madras 600 035, India

First edition 1978
Second edition 1986
Third edition 1992
Reprinted 1993, 1995
Fourth edition 1996

© 1978, 1986, H.K. Lewis: 1992, 1996 Chapman & Hall

Typeset in 9/11pt Times by Mews Photosetting, Beckenham, Kent

Printed in Great Britain by Page Bros. Ltd, Norwich

ISBN 0 412 55560 3

A catalogue record for this book is available from the British Library

Contents

Preface

This edition includes 270 new and revised questions, and the material has been completely rearranged. The questions are based on the text of the 22nd edition of *Bailey & Love's Short Practice of Surgery*, and they are rearranged according to the subjects presented.

A search within the text will reveal the source of the answers, and the student is thereby encouraged to read around the subject presented. In this way the MCQs act as a worthwhile stimulus for the study of surgery.

A.J. Harding Rains
Winchester, April 1996

Instructions

MCQs test your factual knowledge. By using the ones in this book you can test your own progress in learning the principles and practice of surgery.

MCQs are universally used in examinations, and for postgraduate students they are often used as a filter before allowing aspiring candidates to proceed further with other parts of a diploma examination.

Each MCQ is really a series of statements, usually five, and each statement poses a question to you – is it true or is it false? Each statement begins with a stem to which is appended five completions in order to provide five complete statements. Any, or all, can be true. Sometimes none are true.

A useful way to proceed is to read the stem, saying it quietly to yourself, immediately followed by the first suggested completion **A** and then deciding either 'yes', 'true', 'I agree' or 'no', 'false', 'I disagree'. Then proceed similarly with the same stem and the next suggested completion **B**, and so on with **C**, **D** and **E**.

For example:

Stem = **An uncomplicated inguinal hernia**
Completions = **A** has an expansile impulse on coughing.
                  B is reducible.
                  C transilluminates.
                  D can contain bowel.
                  E is best treated by a truss.

Thus, you would say to yourself:
A An uncomplicated inguinal hernia – has an expansile impulse on coughing.
Answer: 'Yes' ('true', 'I agree').
B An uncomplicated inguinal hernia – is reducible.
Answer: 'Yes' ('true', 'I agree').
C An uncomplicated inguinal hernia – transilluminates.
Answer: 'No' ('false', 'I disagree')
D An uncomplicated inguinal hernia – can contain bowel.
Answer 'Yes' (true', 'I agree').
E An uncomplicated inguinal hernia – is best treated by a truss.
Answer: 'No' ('false', 'I disagree').

You score +1 for each correct 'yes' ('true') response. It is also becoming the practice to score +1 each time you give a correct 'no' ('false') response, and –1 for every incorrect response. No points for 'don't know'! Also you are advised not to guess.

By firmly committing yourself to 'yes' and 'no' responses you can score five points for each question, and it follows that you can lose five points.

All the 'yes' answers are at the back of the book and the 'no' responses are therefore obvious.

As stressed in the Preface, explanations for correct and incorrect completions are to be discovered under the appropriate section in your textbook. A few questions are derived from basic medical science knowledge.

Note: It is suggested that if you wish to mark the options you use a soft graphite pencil and not any other writing instrument. In an examination you are given a pencil with which to mark the answer form because usually if a computer is doing the marking it picks up your response via the graphite in the pencil. Try marking the true completions by a vertical line like this | or horizontal —, as these are the ways usually required to mark the computer card. In this book you can erase the responses and start afresh at any time after revision to see if your score improves.

Part One

Questions

Chapter 1

Basic surgical principles
Wounds, tissue repairs, scars
Accident and emergency
Warfare injuries
Acute resuscitation and support
Nutritional support
Pain relief

1. **In the diagnostic component of the surgical process, inspection of an ulcer of the skin confirms that it is**
   - A   an ulcer if there is loss of epithelium.
   - B   malignant if it has undermined edges.
   - C   a squamous carcinoma if it has barely visible pearly edges.
   - D   syphilitic if it has sloping edges.
   - E   likely to be artefacta if of a precise geometric pattern.

2. **The *physical signs* to be sought and checked in relation to a lump or mass include**
   - A   pain.
   - B   throbbing.
   - C   the presence or absence of pulsation.
   - D   ballottement.
   - E   emptying and filling.

3. **The *symptoms* of cellulitis include**
   - A   pain.
   - B   loss of function.
   - C   fluctuation.
   - D   lymphangitis.
   - E   crepitus.

4. **The *physical sign* of crepitus**
   - A   can be elicited when there is subcutaneous emphysema.
   - B   when due to gas infection feels as though the examining hand is palpating a hair mattress.
   - C   is characteristic of cellulitis.
   - D   can be elicited on moving an osteoarthritic joint.
   - E   is elicited by x-ray.

5. **Anatomical imaging is achieved by**
   A   tomography.
   B   magnetic resonance.
   C   employing the Doppler effect.
   D   plethysmography.
   E   urodynamics.

6. **The five cardinal (Celsian) *signs and symptoms* of inflammation include**
   A   pulsation.
   B   fluctuation.
   C   ballottement.
   D   loss of function.
   E   pain.

7. **In the biological process of healing**
   A   platelets are a source of cytokines.
   B   the growth of capillary loops is essential.
   C   fibroblasts synthesise ground substance.
   D   collagen turnover continues for many months.
   E   inflammation necessarily implies infection.

8. **The term 'healing by first intention' means healing by**
   A   using catgut.
   B   obtaining union between two edges of an incision without sub-
        sequent breakdown.
   C   the immediate use of gauze and bandage.
   D   steroid administration.
   E   split skin grafting.

9. **In the healing of a wound, the normal tensile strength of the tissues is generally regained in**
   A   two weeks
   B   six weeks.
   C   six months.
   D   one year
   E   two years

10. **When dealing with**
   A   needlestick injuries to staff, hepatitis immunisation is mandatory.
   B   needlestick injuries to staff, HIV tests should be performed at three and six months.
   C   open injuries to knuckles after a fight, an x-ray is necessary.
   D   injuries due to human bites, neither special treatment nor surveillance is necessary.
   E   abrasion burns, gentle scrubbing in the direction of scratch lines is beneficial.

11. **In the ideal immediate management of incised wounds**
   A   local anaesthesia includes the global use of 1: 10000 adrenaline.
   B   debridement (in the common usage of the word) is employed for every layer.
   C   divided structures should not be repaired at this stage.
   D   wound drainage is unnecessary.
   E   the wound should not be closed.

12. **Wound excision and delayed primary suture**
   A   is applicable only to bullet wounds.
   B   includes excision of all dead tissue.
   C   includes fasciotomy.
   D   leaves the wound wide open after excision.
   E   is essentially the technique of secondary suture.

13. **The extent of tissue damage caused by a bullet depends principally upon**
   A   size.
   B   velocity.
   C   shape.
   D   weight.
   E   consistency.

14. **Muscle damage within a fascial compartment due to a crushing injury**
   A   inevitably results in loss of peripheral pulses.
   B   causes methhaemoglobinaemia.
   C   can cause acute renal failure.
   D   leads to contracture.
   E   is mediated simply by multiple skin incisions.

15. **A decubitus ulcer is**
    A   a venous ulcer.
    B   an ulcer in the region of the elbow.
    C   a pressure sore.
    D   an ulcer of the tongue.
    E   an ulcer without a slough.

16. **Haemorrhage**
    A   is arterial if bright red and spurting in time with the pulse.
    B   is reactionary if occurring four hours after injury.
    C   is secondary if occurring 18 hours after injury.
    D   is dark red if from the pulmonary artery.
    E   from ruptured varicose veins is easily controlled by a tourniquet.

17. **A hypertrophic scar**
    A   is identical to a keloid scar.
    B   requires radiotherapy for a cure.
    C   is a raised red scar which persists for about six months before regressing.
    D   only occurs on the abdomen.
    E   is a premalignant condition.

18. **The true keloid scar**
    A   is considered to be the normal pattern of scar formation.
    B   is common in white-skinned people.
    C   spreads to tissues not affected by the original wound.
    D   tends to get worse even after a year.
    E   can be reduced by steroid preparations.

19. **In the prehospital management of an accident victim, effective care includes**
    A   clearing solid matter from the pharynx.
    B   lifting the mandible forwards.
    C   administering CO_2.
    D   intubating sucking wounds.
    E   applying a tourniquet for lower limb haemorrhage.

20. **The best site for an intramuscular injection is the**
    A   abdomen.
    B   forearm.
    C   inner lower quadrant of the buttock.
    D   outer upper quadrant of the buttock.
    E   front of the thigh.

21. **In road traffic accidents there is a tendency for one type of injury to be associated with another, such as**
   A cervical whiplash with sternal injuries.
   B fracture of lower ribs with ruptured liver.
   C pelvis structure with urinary tract damage.
   D Pott's fracture with ruptured spleen.
   E Le Fort's fractures with dislocated hip.

22. **Injuries characteristically associated with wearing a seat belt include**
   A abdominal wall haematoma.
   B mesenteric laceration.
   C fractured clavicle.
   D fractured pelvis.
   E Monteggia fracture.

23. **Aspects of the Glasgow coma scale which are particularly assessed include**
   A tongue tremor.
   B verbal response.
   C the extensor plantar reflex.
   D motor response.
   E eye opening.

24. **Factors indicating a high risk of multiple injury in motorway accidents include**
   A a flail chest.
   B ejection of the patient.
   C rearward displacement of the front axle.
   D 10% burns.
   E death of another person in the same car.

25. **When a casualty has severe injuries to the face**
   A transport in an ambulance should be in the supine position.
   B an immediate danger to life is blood loss.
   C if there is shock there may be other injuries.
   D an immediate danger is respiratory obstruction due to inhaled blood.
   E if there is bilateral fracture of the jaw the tongue can fall back.

26. **Procedures used in the survey of accident patients include**
   A obtaining a specimen of urine by catheterisation.
   B neck palpation for subcutaneous emphysema.
   C upward traction on the arms for clarity of x-ray of the cervical spine.
   D checking for retropharyngeal haematoma.
   E inspecting the abdominal wall for ecchymosis.

27. **In the assessment of an injury to the head**
    A   the presence of a fractured base is suggested by subconjunctival haemorrhage in which the posterior limit cannot be seen.
    B   the presence of a 'double ring' if blood is dripped on to a sheet indicates a leakage of CSF.
    C   the clotting of blood leaking on to a dressing is observed to be accelerated by the presence of CSF.
    D   deterioration can be due to hypocarbia.
    E   deterioration can be due to hypoperfusion.

28. **In the operative surgery of missile injuries it is essential to**
    A   excise plenty of skin from the wound margin in order to gain access and encourage drainage afterwards.
    B   incise the deep fascia widely.
    C   unite severed nerves.
    D   remove any pieces of bone if part of a comminuted fracture.
    E   pack the wound tightly.

29. **'Delayed primary suture' means**
    A   skin closure of a wound six hours after elective surgery.
    B   skin closure of a wound 18 hours after emergency wound surgery.
    C   the same as secondary suture.
    D   skin closure four to six days after wound surgery if oedema has subsided and tissue is viable.
    E   nerve suture six months after nerve injury.

30. **The serum of a patient with red cell group AB contains**
    A   anti-A and anti-B antibody.
    B   anti-B antibody only.
    C   anti-A antibody only.
    D   no AB antibody.
    E   no Rh factor.

31. **With blast injuries**
    A   the stomach can be perforated.
    B   the caecum can be perforated.
    C   conjunctival haemorrhage can indicate perforation of the globe.
    D   on chest x-ray, opaque fluffiness at the hilum indicates pulmonary oedema.
    E   wound closure is permissible at the end of operations on blast-affected soft tissues.

32. **In replantation surgery of the digits**
    A   the severed digits should be kept in ice.
    B   brachial plexus block is contraindicated.
    C   bone fixation comes first.
    D   dorsal vein anastomosis is performed before volar tendon repair.
    E   priority is given to implantation of the thumb.

33. **The insensible loss of fluid from skin and lungs over 24 hours, in a temperate climate, is normally in the range**
    A   100–250 ml.
    B   250–500 ml.
    C   500–750 ml.
    D   750–1000 ml.
    E   1000–1500 ml.

34. **In the postoperative phase of the surgical patient**
    A   endogenous water released during the oxidation of ingested food amounts to 1000–2000ml in every 24 hours.
    B   small amounts of highly coloured urine with a high specific gravity mean poor renal function.
    C   in pure water depletion the leading sign is oliguria.
    D   a diuresis must be watched for as it means that enough water has been given.
    E   water intoxication is likely when continuous isotonic (5%) dextrose solution is given intravenously.

35. **Sodium depletion**
    A   can be caused by increased secretion of aldosterone.
    B   occurs during the first 48 hours after operation.
    C   can follow prolonged gastric aspiration combined with unlimited ingestion of water.
    D   causes the subcutaneous tissues to feel lax.
    E   results in the urine containing little or no chloride.

36. **Potassium depletion is related to**
    A   increased excretion of potassium for about three to four days postoperatively.
    B   villous tumours of the rectum.
    C   prolonged gastroduodenal aspiration.
    D   muscular spasms.
    E   calculous anuria.

37. **Hypomagnesaemia is associated with**
   A   a serum concentration of 9 mmol/l.
   B   longstanding ulcerative colitis.
   C   small bowel resection.
   D   increased blood pressure.
   E   atrial fibrillation.

38. **Hypokalaemic alkalosis**
   A   is associated with pyloric stenosis.
   B   causes intracellular acidosis.
   C   is indicative of a massive loss of potassium.
   D   can only be reversed rapidly with 60 mmol/l KCl.
   E   requires continuous ECG monitoring during rapid reversal.

39. **Recognised causes of metabolic alkalosis include**
   A   excessive ingestion of absorbable alkali tablets.
   B   repeated vomiting.
   C   Cushing's syndrome.
   D   ulcerative colitis.
   E   starvation.

40. **Ringer's lactate solution contains**
   A   sodium.
   B   potassium.
   C   chlorine.
   D   bicarbonate.
   E   albumin.

41. **Darrow's solution contains**
   A   sodium.
   B   potassium.
   C   chlorine.
   D   bicarbonate.
   E   lactate.

42. **In covert (occult) compensated hypovolaemia, there is characteristically**
   A   no significant reduction of blood pressure.
   B   a significant reduction in splanchnic blood flow.
   C   no reduction in splanchnic blood volume.
   D   thirst.
   E   decreased urinary osmolality.

43. **In overt (open) compensated hypovolaemia, there is characteristically**
   A   bradycardia.
   B   no significant reduction of blood pressure.
   C   warm hands.
   D   a symptomatic positive response to head-down tilt of the body.
   E   a need for high flow oxygen therapy.

44. **In decompensated hypovolaemia due to haemorrhage**
   A   the clinical state is otherwise known as shock.
   B   the vital organs are inadequately perfused.
   C   a thready pulse can be felt.
   D   total circulatory arrest follows if untreated.
   E   blood transfusion must await grouping and cross-matching.

45. **In irreversible shock**
   A   there is multiple organ dysfunction.
   B   the systemic inflammatory response underlies the problem.
   C   tissue hypoxia worsens the situation.
   D   aggressive monitored i.v. therapy is essential.
   E   exotoxins are specifically responsible as being the root cause.

46. **The Systemic Inflammatory Response syndrome (SIRS) is associated with**
   A   tissue oxygen debt.
   B   anaesthesia using nitrous oxide.
   C   cytokine production.
   D   coagulopathy.
   E   supersaturation with vitamin C.

47. **In the measurement of blood loss it is accepted that**
   A   a blood clot the size of a clenched fist is roughly equal to 500 ml.
   B   moderate swelling in a fractured shaft of femur may contain as much as 2000 ml of blood.
   C   total blood and fluid loss during operation is about twice that measured by weighing the swabs in a thoraco-abdominal operation.
   D   blood volume loss can simply be measured by the haematocrit.
   E   blood volume can be measured by monitoring the central venous pressure (CVP)

48. **Features associated with acute blood loss include**
    A restlessness
    B oedema.
    C air hunger
    D tinnitus.
    E blindness.

49. **Measurements of special value in the management of shock include**
    A basal metabolic rate.
    B EEG.
    C pulmonary capillary wedge pressure.
    D haematocrit.
    E urine output.

50. **With reference to the types and features of haemorrhage it can be said that**
    A in arterial haemorrhage the bleeding comes only from the arterial opening nearest the heart.
    B venous haemorrhage from a groin wound requires no more treatment than a pressure dressing for four hours.
    C a 'warning' haemorrhage is characteristic of reactionary haemorrhage.
    D secondary haemorrhage is due to a slipped ligature within 12 hours of operation.
    E a patient with acute blood loss always has a low blood pressure.

51. **The control of bleeding from an incision in the scalp for craniotomy is best achieved by**
    A direct pressure applied to the skin.
    B diathermy to bleeding vessels.
    C eversion of the galea aponeurotica.
    D applying several forceps to the bleeding points.
    E thrombin solution.

52. **After haemorrhage the deficiency of lost plasma proteins is rectified by the**
    A small intestine.
    B liver.
    C spleen.
    D muscles.
    E bone marrow.

53. **In the management of haemorrhage and shock**
    A   morphine is a good drug if given intramuscularly.
    B   simple pyrexial reactions to blood transfusion are usually due to pyrogens.
    C   dextrans are solutions of polysaccharide polymers.
    D   vasoconstrictor drugs should only be given early in treatment.
    E   bacteraemic shock requires vigorous aggressive treatment including blood transfusion and broad spectrum antibiotics.

54. **The complications of blood transfusion include**
    A   sensitisation to leucocytes.
    B   disseminated intravascular coagulation.
    C   Christmas disease.
    D   sickle-cell trait.
    E   immunological sensitisation.

55. **Blood for transfusion should be stored at**
    A   −20°C.
    B   −4°C to 0°C.
    C   +2°C to +6°C.
    D   +10°C to +14°C.
    E   −30°C.

56. **Packed red cells are prepared by**
    A   filtration.
    B   centrifugation.
    C   freeze-drying.
    D   precipitation.
    E   syphoning.

57. **If hepatitis B virus infection is caused by blood transfusion it occurs**
    A   one week later.
    B   six weeks later.
    C   three months later.
    D   six months later.
    E   nine months later.

58. **In an acute emergency if blood has to be given immediately without full laboratory cross-matching it is best to give blood which is**
    A   Group O RhD −ve.
    B   Group O RhD +ve.
    C   Group AB RhD −ve.
    D   Group AB RhD +ve.
    E   Group B RhD + ve.

59. **The methods of assessment of malnutrition in a surgical patient include measurement of**
   A   polymorphonuclear leucocyte number.
   B   the circumference of the thigh.
   C   biceps skin-fold thickness.
   D   serum fibrinogen.
   E   candida skin test.

60. **Factors that operate positively in maintaining the muscle protein of a patient include**
   A   insulin production.
   B   gluconeogenesis by the liver.
   C   cytokine production.
   D   bed-rest.
   E   the hypercatabolic state.

61. **The fat-soluble vitamins include vitamin**
   A   A.
   B   B.
   C   C.
   D   D.
   E   E.

62. **All postoperative patients, after gastric surgery, require**
   A   intravenous alimentation.
   B   2000–4000 calories in 2000–4000 ml of fluid given daily.
   C   high concentrations of carbohydrates i.v.
   D   amino acids taken in at the same time as carbohydrates.
   E   elemental diets.

63. **The recognised unwanted effects of nasogastric tube feeding include**
   A   pulmonary aspiration.
   B   nausea.
   C   diarrhoea.
   D   disturbed liver function.
   E   hyponatraemia.

64. **Feeding by tube enterostomy**
   A   is a form of parenteral nutrition.
   B   is indicated in cases when the passage of a fine bore nasogastric tube is not possible.
   C   is applicable to all cases of intestinal obstruction.
   D   if by gastrostomy the tube should be inserted toward the fundus.
   E   is more satisfactorily accomplished by jejunostomy than by gastrostomy.

65. The local infiltration of an anaesthetic drug

A is ineffective if introduced into an area of infection.
B is contraindicated in any clotting disorder.
C is free from toxic effects.
D with adrenaline (1:200 000) is contraindicated if the patient is taking tricyclic drugs.
E with adrenaline (1:200 000) necessitates a lower dose of anaesthetic drug.

66. Morphine is given for injury primarily because it is

A a sedative.
B an analgesic.
C a diaphoretic.
D an emetic.
E a stimulant.

67. Treatments available for chronic pain includes

A chemical sympathectomy.
B Bier's block.
C nerve stimulation.
D extradural blockade.
E nerve decompression.

Chapter 2

Wound infection
Special infections
Viruses, AIDS
Immunology and transplantation

68. Wound infection is favoured by the presence of
A obesity.
B diabetes.
C jaundice.
D a haematoma.
E dead space.

69. In the local and systemic manifestations of infection of a wound
A sepsis is the systemic manifestation.
B bacteraemia is identical to SIRS.
C cytokines are liberated by Gram-positive bacilli.
D a nosocomial infection is endogenous.
E MSOF is the end point.

70. In cellulitis
A there is non-suppurative invasive infection of the tissues.
B the skin is infiltrated by giant cells.
C spread is characteristic of infection with *Streptococcus pyogenes*.
D tissue destruction is caused by the release of hyaluronidase.
E incision is indicated for Strep. infection.

71. Necrotising fasciitis
A is synonymous with synergistic spreading gangrene.
B is caused by a clostridial infection.
C if affecting the scrotum is called Meleney's gangrene.
D is associated with diabetes insipidus.
E requires aggressive wide excision.

72. Amoebiasis cutis
A is infection of the dermis with *Entamoeba histolytica*.
B tends to be circumscribed.
C is diagnosed simply by slide smear.
D is recognised as a complication of liver abscess.
E readily clears up with steroid therapy.

73. **Of the antibiotics commonly used in surgical practice**
    A   chlorhexidine is effective against Gram-positive organisms.
    B   hexachlorophane acts against Gram-negative organisms.
    C   povidone-iodine in stored solution can allow the proliferation of *Pseudomonas*.
    D   cetrimide is a 10% ethanol solution.
    E   ethyl alcohol is maximally effective as a 70% solution.

74. **The principle organisms of sepsis include**
    A   *Staphylococcus aureus*.
    B   Leishmania.
    C   Nocardia.
    D   *Pseudomonas aeruginosa*.
    E   Bacteroides.

75. **Organisms that are anerobic include**
    A   peptococci.
    B   *Staphylococcus aureus*.
    C   actinomyces.
    D   pneumococci.
    E   bacteroides.

76. **Organisms normally found in the large bowel include**
    A   *Klebsiella*.
    B   *Pseudomonas*.
    C   *Haemophilus*.
    D   *Clostridium difficile*.
    E   *Staphylococcus saprophyticus*.

77. **Factors that favour opportunistic infection of wounds include**
    A   the use of some powerful broad spectrum antibiotics.
    B   irrigation with chlorhexidine solution.
    C   radiotherapy.
    D   prematurity.
    E   burns.

78. **Bacteroides fragilis**
    A   is spore-bearing.
    B   is an aerobe.
    C   colonises the oropharynx.
    D   acts in synergy with MRSA.
    E   is sensitive to the imidazoles.

79. Normally appropriate therapy against a particular organism would be
   A   penicillin against the *Streptococcus*.
   B   tetracycline against *Chlamydia*.
   C   metronidazole against *Staphylococcus aureus*.
   D   ampicillin against *Klebsiella*.
   E   vancomycin against *Clostridium difficile*.

80. An antibioma is
   A   an all-powerful antibiotic.
   B   an antibiotic contaminant.
   C   a malignant tumour caused by an antibiotic.
   D   an excess mass of fibrous tissue around a small abscess persistently treated by antibiotics.
   E   a prescription for an antibiotic.

81. The practice of antisepsis depends entirely upon the use of
   A   carbolic acid.
   B   iodine.
   C   a commitment by surgeons against all infection of wounds caused by trauma or operation.
   D   theatre ventilation.
   E   hexachlorophane.

82. In tetanus infection
   A   the disease is produced by the endotoxin of *Bacillus tetani*.
   B   the toxin travels along nerves to the central nervous system.
   C   the spasm can stop respiration.
   D   a child under the age of one year has an inborn immunity to the disease.
   E   active immunity is conferred by giving ATG (human anti-tetanus globulin).

83. In gas gangrene
   A   a clostridial myositis occurs.
   B   the patient is flushed, pyrexial and drowsy.
   C   a plain x-ray materially helps in the diagnosis.
   D   if the liver becomes affected it is called a 'foaming liver'.
   E   successful treatment is simply blood transfusion and penicillin.

84. **In clostridial pseudomembranous colitis**
   A sloughing of the colonic mucosa occurs.
   B *Cl. difficile* is the organism responsible.
   C cross-reaction of the toxin of *Cl. difficile* with the α–toxin of *Cl. Welchii* produces the respective cytotoxin.
   D the responsible organism cannot be cultured from the stool.
   E treatment is by the use of cephalosporins.

85. **In a tuberculous infection, the organism**
   A is Gram-positive.
   B grows immediately in blood culture.
   C can be tested for drug sensitivity within seven days.
   D with modern treatment is nigh on impossible to eradicate from the body.
   E can be treated with pyrazinamide.

86. **Leprosy**
   A is caused by an organism morphologically akin to the tubercle bacillus.
   B spreads by direct contact and fomites.
   C if of the lepromatous type, forms sharply localised lesions.
   D can manifest a reaction of the Arthus type.
   E therapy includes the use of thalidomide.

87. **Syphilis**
   A is caused by a trepanosome.
   B appears as a primary sore three to four months after infection.
   C is diagnosed in the primary chancre by finding the organisms by dark-field microscopy.
   D in the secondary stage is non-infective as it is an immune response and does not feature the organisms.
   E causes an endarteritis obliterans.

88. **Characteristic features of acquired syphilis include**
   A eighth nerve bilateral deafness.
   B Moon's molars.
   C saddle nose.
   D salmon patches on the cornea.
   E sabre tibia.

89. **The lymph nodes draining a syphilitic chancre of the genitalia area are characteristically**
   A   bulky.
   B   soft.
   C   firm.
   D   cystic.
   E   matted.

90. **Yaws**
   A   is characteristically prevalent in dry desert lands.
   B   is caused by *Treponema pertenue*.
   C   produces serological reactions identical with syphilis.
   D   is a sexually transmitted disease.
   E   occurs primarily on the legs of children.

91. **Candidiasis**
   A   is caused by a yeast.
   B   produces ulcerated raspberry-like swellings (framboesia).
   C   can cause intertrigo.
   D   has a recognised association with AIDS.
   E   is cured with penicillin.

92. **Chancroid (soft sore)**
   A   is caused by Chlamydia.
   B   presents as a beefy red painless ulcer.
   C   is complicated by fluctuant abscesses in the inguinal lymph nodes.
   D   lesions can proceed to phagedaena.
   E   lesions should be excised.

93. **Erysipelas**
   A   is due to infection by MRSA.
   B   declares itself as a vaguely defined rose-pink rash.
   C   causes marked local oedema.
   D   is associated with a mild toxaemia.
   E   responds to penicillin therapy.

94. **A malignant pustule characteristically**
   A   exhibits a central black slough.
   B   has circumferential vesicles.
   C   causes regional lymphadenopathy.
   D   reveals *Aspergillus* on culture.
   E   resolves on incision.

95. **The *Actinomyces israelii* in its pathogenic form**
   A   is an aerobic organism.
   B   is Gram-negative.
   C   is found in abundance in corn and grass.
   D   causes sinus formation.
   E   only submits to prolonged therapy with high dose penicillin.

96. **There is a recognised association between hepatitis B virus infection and**
   A   renal dialysis.
   B   blood transfusion.
   C   needle-stick injuries.
   D   the Dane particle.
   E   amoebiasis.

97. **There is a recognised association between HIV infection and**
   A   lymphadenopathy.
   B   B lymphocytes.
   C   encephalopathy.
   D   Buerger's disease.
   E   *Pneumocystis carinii* infection.

98. **Following infection of the blood with HIV-1 virus there is**
   A   a seroconversion illness with flu-like symptoms and lymph-adenopathy.
   B   a latent period in which the patient remains well but there is a progressive increase in the CD4 positive lymphocyte count.
   C   later, a depletion of immune function which correlates with an increase of the CD4 positive cells.
   D   damage to the thymus.
   E   later, a secretory immune deficiency which occurs in the gut with depletion of IgA-containing jejunal and rectal plasma cells.

99. **Precautions to be taken by the surgeon to prevent contamination with blood infected with HIV-1 virus includes**
   A   wearing boots.
   B   wearing two pairs of surgical gloves.
   C   using a safety mask.
   D   gowning up with a totally waterproof gown.
   E   transferring all sharp instruments between staff via a bowl, never hand-to-hand.

100. **In the event of likely contamination with HIV-1 infected blood by pricking a finger**
   A the finger must be cleaned and washed well in running water immediately.
   B bleeding from the finger should be increased by dependency and venous constriction.
   C hepatitis prophylaxis is necessary.
   D HIV testing is not necessary at this stage.
   E HIV testing is required 12 weeks after contamination.

101. **Major histocompatibility complex (MHC)**
   A is present in the genome of both vertebrates and invertebrates.
   B is located on chromosome 12.
   C products are known as human leucocyte antigens (HLAs)
   D produces membrane proteins that are polymorphic.
   E produces proteins that are used as templates on other cells for the recognition of self.

102. **Cells associated with the immune response include**
   A reticulocytes.
   B oligodendrocytes.
   C dendritic cells.
   D mast cells.
   E Langerhans' cells.

103. **T cells**
   A undergo a selection process for loyalty to self MHC.
   B develop into CD4 and also CD8 types.
   C after apoptosis leave the thymus to join the recirculating pool of immune competent cells.
   D differentiate into plasma cells.
   E are inhibited by the action of reticulocytes.

104. **B cells**
   A are derived from bone marrow.
   B produce antibodies.
   C are precursors of dendritic cells.
   D product cytokines.
   E can be stimulated into clonal expansion by T cells.

105. **In clinical practice, recognised classes of immunoglobulin include Ig**
   A   A.
   B   B.
   C   C.
   D   D.
   E   E.

106. **Cytokines**
   A   are free radicals.
   B   control the proliferation of immunocompetent cells.
   C   act on immune cells via surface receptors.
   D   include those nominated as tumour necrosis factors.
   E   are produced entirely by B cells.

107. **Immunosupressive drugs in common use causing specific major side effects include**
   A   steroids causing bone avascular necrosis.
   B   azathioprine causing gum hyperplasia.
   C   cyclosporine causing thinning of the skin.
   D   antithymocyte globulin causing pulmonary oedema.
   E   antibody OKT3 causing pulmonary oedema.

108. **Guidelines for the diagnosis of brain death include**
   A   the presence of bilateral pinpoint pupils.
   B   no corneal reflex present.
   C   the absence of any effect of sedative drugs.
   D   the agreement of two surgeons expert in transplantation.
   E   the coroner's consent in the case of an accident.

109. **Screening tests on cadaver donors for kidney transplantation include**
   A   ABO blood group compatability.
   B   lymphocyte cross-match.
   C   CMV status
   D   retrograde urography.
   E   bone marrow biopsy.

110. **Procedures useful in determining the cause of oliguria following renal transplantation include**
   A   percutaneous needle biopsy of the kidney.
   B   duplex ultrasonography.
   C   isotope renography.
   D   retrograde urography.
   E   aortography.

111. **The appropriate treatment of surgical complications after renal transplantation includes**
    A   re-exploration for haemorrhage.
    B   re-exploration for ureteric necrosis.
    C   nephrectomy for graft artery thrombosis.
    D   surgical fenestration for lymphocoele.
    E   re-exploration for urinary leak.

112. **The recognised causes of late kidney graft loss include**
    A   a graft rupture.
    B   renal vein thrombosis.
    C   cyclosporine toxicity.
    D   anastomotic dehiscence.
    E   graft neoplasm.

113. **The indications for liver transplantation include**
    A   alcohol abuse.
    B   B hepatitis.
    C   biliary cirrhosis.
    D   drug-induced liver damage.
    E   hydatid cyst.

114. **The management appropriate to surgical complications after liver transplantation would be**
    A   antibiotics for cholangitis.
    B   re-exploration for bile leak.
    C   exploration for preservation damage.
    D   thrombectomy for portal vein thrombosis
    E   thrombectomy for hepatic artery thrombosis.

Chapter 3

Tumours
Cysts
Ulcers
Sinuses
Skin
Burns

115. **A sequestration epithelial dermoid cyst is**
    A   due to squamous cells being driven in by a needle.
    B   due to cells being buried during development.
    C   an example of parthenogenesis.
    D   a sebaceous cyst.
    E   a sarcoma.

116. **Lipomas can be found**
    A   that have undergone saponification.
    B   under the intestinal serosa.
    C   in Dercum's disease.
    D   within the cranium.
    E   which are undergoing carcinomatous change.

117. **Features associated with generalised neurofibromatosis include**
    A   elephantiasis.
    B   plexiform lesions.
    C   cirsoid lesions.
    D   port wine stains.
    E   vitiligo.

118. **Glomus tumours**
    A   are renal tumours.
    B   are cylindromas.
    C   contain neural tissue.
    D   occur in the nail beds.
    E   contain large cuboidal cells.

119. **A hamartoma is**
    A   any collection of blood clot.
    B   a haemorrhagic cyst of the thigh.
    C   a developmental malformation.
    D   a tumour of muscle.
    E   a hepatoma.

120. **Squamous carcinoma**
    A   can occur in transitional cells.
    B   features pallisading of cells.
    C   characteristically arises in a cylindroma.
    D   is manifest in a kerato-acanthoma.
    E   displays acanthosis.

121. **Broder's grading of malignant tumours depends on**
    A   the degree of spread of tumour in the lymphatics.
    B   the degree of differentiation shown by component cells as viewed through the microscope.
    C   a clinical grading for carcinoma of the breast.
    D   an operative grading for carcinoma of the colon.
    E   radiosensitivity.

122. **The seeding of cancer**
    A   gives rise to 'kiss' cancers.
    B   is the reason for transcoelomic spread.
    C   is the cause of Krukenberg's tumours.
    D   occurs in endometriosis.
    E   is the result of metaplasia.

123. **Fibrosarcomas**
    A   are adenomatous.
    B   are mesenchymal.
    C   spread primarily by lymphatic permeation.
    D   occur as an epulis.
    E   are treated by a wide excision with surrounding healthy tissues.

124. **There is a recognised relationship between**
    A   a fibrosarcoma and a scar.
    B   the kangri and an epithelioma.
    C   lupus vulgaris and a rodent ulcer.
    D   the furniture industry and nasopharyngeal carcinoma.
    E   cirrhosis and liver carcinoma.

125. **A false cyst**
    A   has an epithelial lining.
    B   contains exudate.
    C   can form in a haematoma.
    D   arises in an embryonic remnant.
    E   is a characteristic of hydatid cyst.

126. **Conditions recognised to cause trophic ulcers include**
   A   chronic vasospasm.
   B   leprosy.
   C   neurofibromatosis.
   D   diabetes insipidus.
   E   spina bifida.

127. **The manifestations of Leishmania infection include**
   A   Delhi boil.
   B   Baghdad sore.
   C   Singapore ear.
   D   Malta fever.
   E   Lahore sore.

128. **The reasons for the persistence of a sinus or a fistula include the presence of**
   A   a foreign body.
   B   mycobacteria.
   C   Bornholm disease.
   D   anaplastic changes.
   E   marsupialisation.

129. **Guinea worms characteristically**
   A   enter the body through the skin of the abdomen.
   B   procreate in the abdominal connective tissue.
   C   are a cause of sinuses in the lower leg.
   D   use dogs as the alternative host.
   E   cause osteoarthritis.

130. **A sebaceous cyst**
   A   is called as an epidermoid cyst.
   B   only occurs on the face or scalp.
   C   can, if ulcerated, become a sebaceous horn.
   D   characteristically displays a punctum.
   E   if chronically infected is called a Pott's puffy tumour.

131. **A karatin horn**
   A   arises from a sebaceous cyst.
   B   is due to matting of hair.
   C   is a papilloma with excess keratin formation.
   D   is congenital.
   E   is a molluscum sebaceum.

132. **The molluscum sebaceum is**
    - A a sebaceous cyst.
    - B called Bowen's disease.
    - C an epithelioma.
    - D a keratoacanthoma.
    - E known to heal spontaneously.

133. **Dermatofibrosarcoma protuberans**
    - A occurs most commonly on the extremities.
    - B is composed of interwoven bands of fibroblasts.
    - C arises in scar tissue some years after the scar has developed.
    - D begins as a painless nodule.
    - E frequently metastasises.

134. **Granuloma pyogenicum should be treated definitively by**
    - A cauterisation.
    - B antibiotic ointment.
    - C excision.
    - D radiotherapy.
    - E incision.

135. **A rhinophyma is a**
    - A sebaceous cyst of the nose.
    - B rodent ulcer of the nose.
    - C glandular form of acne rosacea.
    - D nasal form of Boeck's sarcoid.
    - E hard skin pad on the sole of the foot.

136. **A port wine stain (naevus flammeus) is a**
    - A premalignant lesion of the skin.
    - B type of melanoma.
    - C type of bruising of the skin.
    - D type of haemangioma.
    - E tattoo.

137. **A strawberry angioma 1 cm × 1 cm on the forearm of a neonate should be managed by using**
    - A cryosurgery.
    - B radiotherapy.
    - C excision.
    - D masterly inactivity.
    - E electrocoagulation.

138. Premalignant conditions of the skin itself include
A Bowen's disease.
B leucoplakia.
C solar keratosis.
D acanthosis nigricans.
E cylindroma.

139. Marjolin's ulcer characteristically
A is an adenocarcinoma.
B develops rapidly in scar tissue.
C is painful.
D does not, in the first instance, spread to regional lymph nodes.
E complicates hidradenitis suppurativa.

140. A basal cell carcinoma of the skin
A histologically exhibits intercellular bridging.
B is radioresistant.
C characteristically metastasises to the regional lymph nodes.
D most commonly occurs at the outer canthus of the eye.
E can, if small, be treated successfully by cryosurgery.

141. The types of basal cell carcinoma of the skin include the
A cystic.
B pigmented.
C morphoeic.
D field fire.
E pyogenic granuloma.

142. Squamous cell carcinoma of the skin characteristically affects or appears in
A children.
B areas of lupus erythematosus.
C skin exposed to sunbathing many years previously.
D vitiligous skin with an increased frequency compared with normal skin.
E the albinos of dark-skinned races.

143. Squamous cell carcinoma of the skin
A histologically exhibits keratinisation.
B histologically exhibits pallisading of cells.
C can occur in longstanding hidradenitis suppurativa.
D if situated at the angle of the mouth tends to metastasise early to submandibular lymph nodes.
E is radioresistant.

144. **The blue naevus**
    A   is a type of vascular hamartoma.
    B   is so called because the melanocytes contain blue pigment.
    C   develops a melanotic halo.
    D   occurs only on the face.
    E   is characteristically benign.

145. **Types of malignant melanoma with characteristic features include**
    A   the spreading superficial type, which is the commonest and has an irregular edge.
    B   the melanotic freckle, which is very malignant.
    C   the nodular type which ulcerates and bleeds.
    D   the acral-lentiginous type, which occurs chiefly on the dorsum of the hands and the feet.
    E   the amelanotic type, which does not metastasise.

146. **A malignant melanoma characteristically**
    A   only arises in a pre-existing pigmented naevus.
    B   is common before puberty.
    C   may be surrounded by a halo.
    D   may be both melanotic and amelanotic.
    E   spreads by the lymphatics and not by the blood stream.

147. **Acceptable management of a malignant melanoma (stage 1) of the skin of the lower leg includes**
    A   excision biopsy with surrounding 2 cm of skin.
    B   with biopsy excision, the removal of underlying deep fascia.
    C   cryosurgery without biopsy.
    D   prophylactic isolated limb perfusion with melphalan.
    E   prophylactic radical block dissection of regional lymph nodes in the groin.

148. **Kaposi's angiosarcoma**
    A   is derived from capillaries.
    B   is associated with lymphoma.
    C   is associated with malaria.
    D   can run its course in other organs without skin manifestations.
    E   commonly begins on the feet.

149. **A partial thickness burn**
   A   is sensitive.
   B   can become a full thickness burn.
   C   will separate as a slough in two to three weeks.
   D   requires a split skin graft.
   E   is likely to benefit from tangential excision.

150. **The treatment of burns includes**
   A   irrigation with cold water in first aid.
   B   exposure.
   C   encouraging the formation of a good scab.
   D   excision and grafting.
   E   the application of silver sulphadiazine ointment.

151. **The management of a patient with a burn of 30% of the body surface includes**
   A   the use of morphine i.m.
   B   blood transfusion.
   C   dextran i.v.
   D   haematocrit readings.
   E   monitoring urine output.

152. **Acceptable surgical procedures for the treatment of a 10 cm diameter deep burn on the back of the leg includes**
   A   awaiting desloughing and performing secondary suture.
   B   using a split skin graft as a dressing, stat.
   C   excision and applying a split skin graft.
   D   excision and using a flap graft.
   E   performing tangential excision and applying a split skin graft under tourniquet control.

Chapter 4

Arterial disorders
Venous disorders
Lymphatics and lymph nodes

153. **'Rest pain' occurs**
   A anywhere in the body at rest.
   B in the thigh of a patient with Buerger's disease.
   C in the calf of a patient with intermittent claudication.
   D in the foot of a patient with severe vascular disease.
   E in the back.

154. **Harvey's sign is the**
   A loss of hair from the toes in peripheral vascular disease.
   B distended veins in the foot in spite of arterial occlusion.
   C gauging of the speed of venous return by emptying the length of vein.
   D transmitted pressure wave on coughing in severe varicose veins.
   E presence of petechiae in the antecubital fossa in scarlet fever.

155. **The term ischaemia means**
   A pain in the ischial tuberosities.
   B anaemia due to malignant secondaries in the ischial part of the pelvis.
   C lack of blood flow.
   D increased blood flow.
   E polycythaemia.

156. **In a patient with severe peripheral vascular disease of the legs**
   A rest pain is felt in the calf muscles.
   B rest pain is relieved by elevation.
   C hot foot baths are beneficial for cold feet.
   D sympathectomy cannot be of any value.
   E glycosuria is relevant.

157. **Methods used to investigate arterial disease include**
   A auscultation.
   B duplex imaging.
   C angioplasty.
   D digital subtraction angiography.
   E myelography.

158. **A Seldinger needle is used for**
   A   liver biopsy.
   B   suturing skin.
   C   arteriography.
   D   lymphography.
   E   breast biopsy.

159. **A contraindication to elective arterial bypass operations is evidence of**
   A   diabetes
   B   heart failure.
   C   Paget's disease.
   D   coronary thrombosis six months previously.
   E   pyelonephritis

160. **Operations of proven value for intermittent claudication include**
   A   lumbar sympathectomy.
   B   obturator neurectomy.
   C   thrombo-endarterectomy.
   D   deep vein ligation.
   E   vein bypass graft.

161. **In arterial surgery the best vein to use for bypass is the**
   A   cephalic.
   B   femoral.
   C   long saphenous.
   D   short saphenous.
   E   popliteal.

162. **Operations of value for an obliterated lower abdominal aorta include**
   A   endarterectomy.
   B   vein bypass graft.
   C   excision of the aorta.
   D   femorofemoral cross-over graft.
   E   aortofemoral Dacron bifurcation graft.

163. **Thromboendarterectomy is**
   A   the ideal operation for Buerger's disease.
   B   the ideal operation for Raynaud's disease.
   C   used for carotid artery stenosis.
   D   the same operation as embolectomy.
   E   a graft technique.

164. The femoral artery in the upper part of the femoral triangle
A   is a continuation of the internal iliac artery.
B   is crossed by the superficial circumflex iliac vein.
C   lies medial to the common femoral vein.
D   has the femoral nerve on its medial side.
E   is separated from the hip joint by the tendon of psoas major.

165. The presence of an embolus in a limb is recognised by there being
A   complete loss of feeling.
B   hyperaemia of the whole limb.
C   hyperaesthesia of the whole limb.
D   the presence of Brown-Séquard's syndrome.
E   a proximal water-hammer pulse.

166. A Fogarty catheter is designed to be used for
A   intravenous (parenteral) nutrition.
B   ureteric catheterisation.
C   removing blood clots from arteries.
D   arteriography.
E   draining the bladder.

167. Fat embolism is associated with
A   multiple fractures.
B   necrotising fasciitis.
C   petechial haemorrhages.
D   adipectomy.
E   ECT.

168. Materials used in therapeutic embolism include
A   blood clot.
B   gel foam sponge.
C   balloons.
D   stainless steel coils.
E   ethyl alcohol.

169. With injury to a main limb artery from any cause
A   intimal tears lead to distal embolism.
B   penetrating wounds not precisely attended to are likely to be followed by A-V fistula.
C   a vein from the affected limb is very handy for use as an inter-position graft.
D   fractures, if present and alongside, must be stabilised.
E   absence of distal pulses after arterial repair is most likely due to spasm.

34

170. **The local management of gangrene of the foot includes**
    A   daily foot baths.
    B   heat by a heat pad.
    C   cooling by ice.
    D   minor surgical toilet.
    E   the use of a sheepskin.

171. **In a diabetic ischaemic foot**
    A   infection spreads upwards by the subfascial planes.
    B   a plain x-ray of the foot is mandatory.
    C   rest pain is troublesome.
    D   an above knee amputation of the leg is the likely outcome.
    E   a neuropathic ankle joint is likely to be present.

172. **Bedsores are**
    A   predisposed to by hypovolaemia.
    B   predisposed to by wrinkled bedsheets.
    C   are to be expected if erythema appears and does not change colour on pressure.
    D   related to indisciplined patient care.
    E   unlikely if the site at risk is protected by the application of Opsite.

173. **Frostbite of the toes and foot**
    A   is not uncommon in the homeless.
    B   includes blistering, swelling and gangrene as clinical features.
    C   should be managed immediately with a hot-water bottle or heat pad.
    D   should be rubbed with a dry towel.
    E   means that an above knee amputation will be mandatory.

174. **Trench foot is**
    A   sodden infected skin of the foot following the digging of a trench in wet weather.
    B   an ischaemic condition of the foot following exposure to damp and cold in tight footwear.
    C   gas gangrene of the foot.
    D   chilblains of the toes.
    E   a fungus infection.

175. **Ainhum is a lesion which is**
   A   a type of anal fissure.
   B   a fibromatous polyp at the anal margin.
   C   mycotic infection of the heel.
   D   a fibrotic process affecting a toe.
   E   a perianal sinus.

176. **In amputation of the leg, the stump**
   A   should be a conical stump.
   B   length should be not less than 20 cm if above the knee.
   C   length should preferably be 10–12 cm if below the knee.
   D   flaps can be skew.
   E   in a Syme amputation includes a sliver of calcaneum.

177. **In the management of amputation phantom pain, it is advisable to**
   A   reassure the patient that the feeling of a painful phantom limb will disappear in time.
   B   proceed with postamputation exercises.
   C   proceed with limb fitting.
   D   explain phantom pain to students and nurses in front of the patient.
   E   amputate at a higher level.

178. **The commonest cause of a true aneurysm is**
   A   congenital.
   B   syphilitic.
   C   atherosclerosis.
   D   a gunshot wound.
   E   an arteriovenous shunt for dialysis.

179. **Regarding aneurysms**
   A   a saccular aneurysm is a false aneurysm.
   B   an arteriovenous aneurysm is always congenital in origin.
   C   expansile pulsation is an extrinsic sign of aneurysm.
   D   gangrene is an intrinsic sign of an aneurysm.
   E   an aneurysm may be mistaken for an abscess.

180. **If a child aged 10 has a congenital arteriovenous fistula in the region of the knee joint**
    A   the veins are collapsed.
    B   the leg of the affected side tends to be shorter than that on the unaffected side.
    C   the cardiac output is decreased.
    D   ulceration of the leg above the ankle can occur.
    E   it can be cured by ligation of the feeding artery.

181. **Patients with abdominal aortic aneurysm**
    A   if symptomatic will all be dead in a year.
    B   if symptomatic should all have surgery.
    C   if asymptomatic with a 5 cm diameter aneurysm carry a 75% chance of rupture.
    D   if asymptomatic can carry a 2–5% mortality if operated upon electively.
    E   are able to have the diameter of the sac measured by aortography.

182. **Popliteal aneurysm**
    A   is usually due to syphilis.
    B   accounts for 70% of all peripheral aneurysms.
    C   is most commonly unilateral.
    D   is associated with an abdominal aortic aneurysm in one-third of cases.
    E   can be repaired without total excision.

183. **Temporal arteritis is**
    A   a local collagen disease.
    B   a feature of Takayasu's arteriopathy.
    C   a variety of Buerger's disease.
    D   associated with blindness.
    E   confirmed by surgical biopsy.

184. **A patient who is beginning to suffer from Buerger's disease (thrombo-angiitis obliterans)**
    A   has scleroderma.
    B   is likely to be a woman.
    C   is always an Ashkenazi Jew.
    D   suffers from atherosclerosis.
    E   could get gangrene of the bowel.

185. **A man aged 50 suffers from unilateral Raynaud's phenomenon in the hand. Recognised associations include**
   A   Raynaud's disease.
   B   atherosclerosis of the subclavian artery.
   C   Buerger's disease.
   D   cervical rib.
   E   infective bacterial endocarditis.

186. **Lumbar sympathectomy is of value in the management of**
   A   intermittent claudication.
   B   distal ischaemia affecting the skin of the toes.
   C   arteriovenous fistula.
   D   diabetic neuropathy.
   E   back pain.

187. **Chemical sympathectomy is effected by using**
   A   5% phenol solution in arachis oil.
   B   10% phenol solution in olive oil.
   C   12% phenol in water.
   D   5% phenol solution in water.
   E   2% phenol in dextran.

188. **In lumbar sympathectomy the sympathetic chain in its usual position is likely to be confused with the**
   A   ureter.
   B   psoas minor.
   C   genitofemoral nerve.
   D   ilioinguinal nerve.
   E   lymphatics.

189. **The nerve of Kuntz is an important landmark in**
   A   lumbar sympathectomy.
   B   cervicodorsal sympathectomy.
   C   obturator neurectomy.
   D   splanchnicectomy.
   E   herniorrhaphy.

190. **The term 'venous pump' refers to**
   A   the apparatus used for rapid transfusion of blood.
   B   part of autotransfusion apparatus.
   C   the left atrium.
   D   the presence of valves in the inferior vena cava.
   E   the musculofascial anatomy and physiology of the calf.

191. **Investigations of value in venous disorders include**
   A   ventriculography.
   B   duplex imaging.
   C   Doppler studies.
   D   plethysmography.
   E   Perthe's test.

192. **Venous thrombosis is associated with**
   A   muscular violence.
   B   anti-thrombin III deficiency.
   C   domicile in equatorial countries.
   D   visceral neoplasm.
   E   polycythaemia vera.

193. **The types of venous thrombosis include**
   A   Leriche's syndrome.
   B   phlegmasia caerulea dolens.
   C   Takayasu's disease.
   D   mesenteric.
   E   venous gangrene.

194. **The prevention of venous thrombosis in relation to a major operation includes**
   A   pneumatic calf compression.
   B   the use of graduated compression stockings.
   C   the use of Esmark's bandage.
   D   the use of low molecular weight heparin.
   E   the infusion of isotonic saline.

195. **Heparin overdose can be managed effectively by**
   A   giving prostaglandins.
   B   giving steroids.
   C   stopping any further administration of the substance.
   D   giving protamine sulphate.
   E   giving prostigmine.

196. **A white leg is due to**
   A   femoral deep vein thrombosis.
   B   lymphatic obstruction.
   C   femoral vein thrombosis and lymphathic obstruction.
   D   vena cava thrombosis.
   E   femoral embolus.

197. **Axillary vein thrombosis**
    A   is associated with DIY activities.
    B   gives a positive Homan's sign.
    C   causes pain in the forearm.
    D   is a recognised cause of Raynaud's phenomenon.
    E   can be limited by early anticoagulant therapy.

198. **Varicose veins occurring before the age of 20 are recognised to be associated with**
    A   Perthe's disease.
    B   extensive cavernous haemangioma.
    C   acquired arteriovenous fistula.
    D   congenital arterial arteriovenous fistula.
    E   Buerger's disease.

199. **The clinical assessment of varicose veins includes the use of**
    A   Hess's test.
    B   the Brodie-Trendelenburg test.
    C   Perthe's test.
    D   duplex imaging.
    E   the muscle-stretch test.

200. **Clinically a saphena varix is most likely to be confused with a**
    A   Baker's cyst.
    B   femoral hernia.
    C   spermatocele.
    D   soft sore.
    E   varicocele.

201. **The Brodie-Trendelenburg test is used to detect**
    A   the presence of deep femoral vein thrombosis.
    B   the integrity of the long saphenous nerve.
    C   the presence of an incompetent valve at the saphenofemoral junction.
    D   the presence of an incompetent valve at the junction of the short saphenous and popliteal veins.
    E   CDH.

202. **If a female patient aged 30 presents with the sudden recent appearance of varicose veins of the leg, one is wise to**
   - A   look for a saphena varix.
   - B   perform a rectal examination.
   - C   perform an abdominal examination.
   - D   advise operation.
   - E   consider Milroy's disease as a cause.

203. **The treatment of varicose veins of the legs includes**
   - A   injection of 5 ml of phenol in arachis oil into the veins.
   - B   injection of ethanolamine oleate 5%.
   - C   hot baths.
   - D   ligature of the common femoral vein.
   - E   stripping the superficial femoral vein.

204. **Operations for varicose veins are best accomplished by**
   - A   stripping.
   - B   multiple subcutaneous ligatures.
   - C   subfascial ligatures.
   - D   division and ligation at the sites of a bad leak from the deep to the superficial venous system.
   - E   injecting sclerosants throughout.

205. **Venous ulcers are associated with**
   - A   superficial venous valve insufficiency.
   - B   deep venous valve insufficiency.
   - C   microthrombosis.
   - D   syphilis.
   - E   talipes equinus-like deformity.

206. **Factors implicated in the aetiology of venous ulceration include**
   - A   venous hypertension.
   - B   slowing of blood in the capillaries.
   - C   trapping of white cells.
   - D   free radical damage.
   - E   the presence of Dopplerite.

207. The management of a venous ulcer (after Bisgaard) includes
    A   curettage of the ulcer.
    B   the application of spirally applied elastic bandaging.
    C   active movements to the calf muscles in elevation.
    D   teaching correct walking, heel down first.
    E   massage to the indurated area around the ulcer.

208. Acute lymphangitis
    A   is a common feature of mild bacterial infection.
    B   is usually due to infection with *Streptococcus viridans*.
    C   can bypass the lymph nodes immediately draining the site of
         infection.
    D   should be investigated by emergency lymphangiography.
    E   should be incised without delay and culture swabs taken.

209. Lymphangiography of the leg is performed by
    A   an injection of sodium diatrizoate subcutaneously between the toes.
    B   injecting sodium diatrizoate retrogradely under pressure into a
         small vein on the dorsum of the foot.
    C   dissecting lymphatics through an incision on the dorsum of the foot.
    D   outlining the lymphatics by a subcutaneous injection of the leg
         above the ankle with patent blue dye.
    E   the use of an infusion pump.

210. Finding the cause of unilateral lymphoedema of the leg includes
    A   taking a family history.
    B   looking for chronic infection of the foot.
    C   looking for early malignant disease.
    D   looking for filariasis.
    E   performing a Casoni test.

211. Milroy's disease characteristically is lymphoedema that
    A   follows filariasis.
    B   is familial.
    C   follows erysipelas.
    D   is the sequel to 'white leg'.
    E   is due to malignant disease.

212. A cystic hygroma is a
    A   type of hydrocele.
    B   type of lymphangioma.
    C   type of brachial cyst.
    D   cystic sweat gland tumour.
    E   cystic rodent.

213. **Filariasis**
    A   is caused by a cestode worm.
    B   is spread by one of the anopheles group of mosquito.
    C   can be diagnosed on a nocturnal blood smear.
    D   causes chylous reflux.
    E   causes elephantiasis neuromatosa.

214. **Tuberculous lymphadenitis**
    A   does not occur in the aged.
    B   can be caused by drinking infected milk.
    C   displays the presence of Reed-Sternberg cells on histological examination.
    D   as a rule causes discrete rubbery lymph nodes.
    E   is the originator of scrofulous dermatitis (the King's Evil).

215. **The histological appearance of Hodgkin's lymphoma includes the presence of**
    A   Langerhans' cells.
    B   eosinophils.
    C   reticulum cells.
    D   Hassall's corpuscles.
    E   acanthotic cells.

216. **Procedures currently helpful in the assessment of lymphoma include**
    A   chest x-ray.
    B   intravenous urography.
    C   full laparotomy.
    D   tonsillectomy.
    E   block dissection of glands of the neck.

217. **Simple steps in the diagnosis of a solitary swelling in the left anterior triangle of the neck of a young person include**
    A   examination of the tonsils
    B   a white cell count.
    C   an x-ray of the chest.
    D   an excision biopsy of the swelling under local anaesthetic.
    E   incision of the swelling.

218. There is a recognised close association between

    A   Hodgkin's lymphoma and Langerhans' giant cells.

    B   Boeck's sarcoid and Reed-Sternberg cells.

    C   cysticerosis and calcification.

    D   amyloid disease and sepsis.

    E   gonorrhoea and acute arthritis of the knee.

Chapter 5

Fractures and dislocations

219. **In the stages of healing of a fracture of tubular bone, according to the haematoma theory,**
A   the haematoma is invaded by granulation tissue.
B   acanthosis occurs.
C   macrophages remove the haematoma.
D   the repair includes the formation of fibrocartilagenous tissue.
E   callus is distributed throughout the area occupied by the fracture haematoma.

220. **In the stages of healing of a fracture of tubular bone, according to the periosteal (proliferative) theory,**
A   osteogenic cells are stimulated to proliferate within hours of the fracture occurring.
B   callus collars are formed around each fragment.
C   the callus collars grow toward each other.
D   squamous metaplasia occurs.
E   osteogenic cells become osteoblasts.

221. **Fracture callus characteristically**
A   exhibits bony trabeculae cemented to the shaft.
B   exhibits an outer layer of chondrocytes.
C   includes a V-shaped cartilagenous formation.
D   is cemented to the original cortex.
E   becomes Haversian bone.

222. **A compound fracture**
A   is present if a laceration of mucous membrane connects with the fracture haematoma.
B   is inevitably present if a laceration of the skin overlies a spiral fracture of the humerus.
C   can be present if skin death from ischaemia overlies a fractured tibia.
D   is not a cause of septicaemia.
E   if compound from without carries a poorer prognosis than a compound fracture from within.

223. **Fracture lines can be described as being**
   A   comminuted.
   B   butterfly.
   C   spiral.
   D   compression.
   E   twisted.

224. **The names given to the displacement in a fracture of a long bone include**
   A   angulation.
   B   shift.
   C   twist.
   D   distraction.
   E   subluxation.

225. **At the stage of clinical union of a fracture of tubular bone**
   A   the bone bridging the fracture has a normal radiological appearance.
   B   unprotected stress can lead to re-fracture.
   C   local palpation produces little or no tenderness.
   D   consolidation has occurred.
   E   the swelling at the fracture site has disappeared.

226. **The recognised causes of delayed union include**
   A   compound fracture.
   B   infection.
   C   ankylosis.
   D   uraemia.
   E   distraction.

227. **Union of a simple uncomplicated transverse fracture of the tibia in an adult normally takes**
   A   six weeks.
   B   eight weeks.
   C   12 weeks.
   D   18 weeks.
   E   26 weeks.

228. **Malunion of a fracture is**
   A   a fracture which unites in a position of deformity.
   B   delayed union of a fracture.
   C   non-union of a fracture.
   D   followed by pseudoarthrosis.
   E   due to tuberculosis.

229. **Fractures which do not impact include**
 A   fracture of the vault of the skull.
 B   a compression fracture.
 C   a simple fracture.
 D   a transverse fracture of the patella.
 E   fracture of the neck of the femur.

230. **The causes of non-union of a fracture include**
 A   very slight bending movements during the healing phase.
 B   infection of the fracture haematoma.
 C   anoxia.
 D   uraemia.
 E   Paget's disease (osteitis deformans).

231. **Practical schemes for the management of fractures include**
 A   treating the patient specifically according to the radiographic appearance.
 B   reduction by gravity.
 C   clinical manipulation.
 D   open operation.
 E   the use of external fixators.

232. **As an alternative to plaster of Paris, a tubular bone fracture can be stabilised by**
 A   external skeletal fixators.
 B   compression plating.
 C   osteoclasis.
 D   skin traction.
 E   intramedullary nailing.

233. **In the management of compound fractures the guidelines include the fact that**
 A   it is a surgical emergency.
 B   treatment aims at sterilising the fracture site.
 C   a tourniquet should be used if possible to help the surgeon examine the site.
 D   the wound should be closed at once in order to prevent secondary infection.
 E   while the skin is healing the fracture cannot be splinted in plaster.

234. **Operative stabilisation of a tubular bone fracture is of recognised value for**
    A   replacing small fragments adjacent to joints.
    B   fractures of the patella.
    C   patients with a head injury.
    D   repair of a main artery to a limb.
    E   those occurring in infants.

235. **Characteristic features of acute compartment syndrome in the lower leg include**
    A   gross swelling.
    B   normal pulses.
    C   normal sensation distally.
    D   acute pain on employing the stretch test.
    E   venous occlusion.

236. **Early complications of lower limb fractures include**
    A   blisters.
    B   gas gangrene.
    C   fat embolism.
    D   osteoarthritis.
    E   Friedreich's ataxia.

237. **Recognised late complications of fractures include**
    A   Dupuytrens's contracture.
    B   hypertrophic non-union.
    C   Sudeck's atrophy.
    D   myositis ossificans.
    E   osteitis fibrosa cystica.

238. **Fractures occurring in children differ from those in adults in the following respects. In children**
    A   the fractures unite more slowly.
    B   malunion can be partly corrected by growth.
    C   joint stiffness is common after immobilisation.
    D   immobilisation by splinting is the method of choice in treatment.
    E   involvement of the epiphyseal plate is uncommon as the plate is stronger than the bone.

239. **Recognised features of fractures involving the growth plate and epiphysis in children include**
   A   greenstick fractures.
   B   end-on crushes.
   C   intra-articular fractures.
   D   butterfly fractures.
   E   a fracture line that runs through part of the growth plate lying between calcified and uncalcified cartilage.

240. **With injury and fracture of articular cartilage**
   A   true healing does not occur.
   B   the defect is filled with fibrocartilage.
   C   muscle wasting surrounding the joint is unusual.
   D   locking can occur.
   E   blood within the joint will not clot.

241. **A march fracture**
   A   is a feature of effort syndrome.
   B   may not show up on immediate x-ray.
   C   is the result of localised stress and fatigue.
   D   in the foot is predisposed to by a short first metatarsal.
   E   is a vernal condition.

242. **Specifically diagnostic of a joint ligament rupture is**
   A   local tenderness.
   B   pain when ligament is stressed.
   C   bruising.
   D   local swelling.
   E   mechanical instability.

243. **With a midshaft fracture of the clavicle**
   A   the coraco-acromial ligament is ruptured.
   B   significant displacement of the bone ends is common.
   C   the fracture should be reduced.
   D   malunion is uncommon.
   E   non-union is possible.

244. **A fracture of the midshaft of the clavicle is best treated by**
   A   clavicle rings.
   B   a figure-of-eight bandage.
   C   open reduction and plating.
   D   an intramedullary nail.
   E   a broad arm sling and analgesics.

245. If a patient presents with an acromioclavicular dislocation

A the coracoclavicular ligament has also ruptured.

B the clavicle is held in place by the clavipectoral fascia.

C reduction is best maintained by a temporary screw through the clavicle to engage in the coracoid process.

D it is acceptable merely to rest the arm in a sling and to mobilise the shoulder when the pain has settled.

E the late sequel of osteoarthrosis can be treated by excision of the outer end of the clavicle.

246. In dislocation of the shoulder

A the injury is produced by a fall with the arm fully abducted.

B the commonest position for the head of the humerus to move into is subspinous.

C the axillary nerve (circumflex) is likely to be damaged.

D Kocher's method of reduction is no longer necessary.

E the easiest method of reduction is by simple pressure if a carefully administered general anaesthetic with a short-acting muscle relaxant is given.

247. With fractures of the proximal humerus

A the injury is through the anatomical neck characteristically following a fall on the outstretched hand.

B fracture of the surgical neck is common in the elderly.

C fracture of the anatomical neck may be combined with anterior dislocation of the shoulder.

D fracture of the surgical neck is treated by the excision of the head of the humerus and replacement by a prosthesis.

E fracture of the anatomical neck with dislocation of the shoulder is best treated by rest in a sling with active mobilisation once pain has subsided.

248. Complications of fracture of the proximal humerus include

A paralysis of the deltoid muscle.

B numbness of skin over a small area of the deltoid.

C avascular necrosis of the head of the humerus.

D non-union.

E tardy ulnar palsy.

249. **In fracture of the shaft of the humerus**
   A   a butterfly fragment may be present.
   B   the fracture should be reduced under an anaesthetic.
   C   the arm should be held by plaster abducted to 60° on a traction frame secured to the body.
   D   radial palsy is a complication.
   E   pseudoarthrosis is common.

250. **Concerning supracondylar fracture of the humerus in a child**
   A   the injury is caused by a fall on the point of the elbow.
   B   the displacement includes forward displacement of the distal fragment.
   C   the elbow swells rapidly.
   D   ischaemia of the forearm and hand is a distinct possibility.
   E   after reduction the child may be allowed to go home provided he or she attends the fracture clinic the next day.

251. **Regarding a fracture of the medial epicondyle of the humerus**
   A   it is an avulsion injury.
   B   the fragment of bone may be rotated.
   C   the fragment of bone fortunately does not enter the elbow joint.
   D   a rotated fragment requires operative re-attachment to the epicondyle.
   E   active and passive movements of the elbow joint should begin as soon as possible.

252. **Myositis ossificans**
   A   occurs only at the elbow.
   B   only follows a fracture.
   C   is ossification in a haematoma.
   D   is bone formation between rather than in muscles.
   E   is discouraged by early active exercises to the part.

253. **Dislocation of the elbow**
   A   occurs from falling on the point of the elbow.
   B   is commonly a posterolateral dislocation.
   C   can include divergent dislocation of the radius and ulna.
   D   can include fracture of the coronoid.
   E   is best managed by active exercises commenced 48 hours after reduction.

254. **Among the features and types of forearm fractures**
   A   a fractured shaft of ulna with dislocation of the inferior radioulnar joint is a Monteggia fracture.
   B   a fractured shaft of radius with dislocation of the superior radioulnar joint is a Galeazzi fracture.
   C   remodelling will correct any residual rotational problem.
   D   synostosis can occur.
   E   acute compartmental syndrome is a complication.

255. **Bennett's fracture is a**
   A   reversed Colles' fracture.
   B   fracture of the scaphoid bone in the wrist.
   C   fracture of the radial styloid (chauffeur's fracture).
   D   fracture dislocation of the first metacarpal.
   E   cause of mallet finger.

256. **In a Colles's fracture the distal fragment is**
   A   displaced dorsally.
   B   rotated dorsally.
   C   displaced medially.
   D   rotated medially.
   E   pronated.

257. **Problems following reduction of a Colles' fracture include**
   A   the backward angulation of the distal fragment.
   B   recurrent displacement of the inferior radioulnar joint.
   C   carpal tunnel syndrome.
   D   rupture of the tendon of the flexor pollicis longus.
   E   algodystrophy.

258. **In fractures of the waist of the scaphoid**
   A   the patients are typically thin elderly women.
   B   the clinical features suggest a diagnosis of a sprained wrist.
   C   there is tenderness in the anatomical snuff-box.
   D   an A-P and a lateral x-ray of the wrist should show the fracture line immediately.
   E   the fracture is treated in a plaster for two weeks then the plaster is removed and the wrist mobilised.

259. With mallet finger

A the injury is due to a direct blow to the distal interphalangeal joint.

B there is commonly a comminuted fracture of the distal phalanx.

C the distal phalanx is held in 30° flexion.

D passive extension is impossible.

E the deformity often persists in spite of treatment.

260. Accident victims

A must have an x-ray of the pelvis if there is pain on stressing the pelvis.

B with a fracture outside the pelvic ring are managed by bed-rest until the symptoms settle.

C with a single ring pelvis fracture are managed by bed-rest until the symptoms settle.

D with a double ring fracture of the pelvis need skeletal traction and pelvic sling for six to eight weeks.

E if male with pubic rami fractures suffer extreme scrotal ecchymosis.

261. Complications of pelvic fractures include

A blood loss.

B bladder injuries.

C DVT.

D malunion.

E bowel entrapment.

262. In posterior dislocation of the hip

A the leg is flexed.

B the leg is abducted.

C the leg is externally rotated.

D reduction is usually easy.

E 50% of dislocations are followed by avascular necrosis of the femoral head if there is delay in reduction.

263. Intracapsular fractures of the neck of the femur

A always occur in elderly women and men.

B may be impacted in abduction.

C when unimpacted are recognised by a shortened leg that lies in external rotation.

D are invariably operated on.

E if unimpacted are unlikely to be followed by non-union.

264. **If a patient has avascular necrosis of the head of the femur**
   A   the head has firstly been infarcted.
   B   the infarct is painful.
   C   steroid therapy may be a cause.
   D   irradiation is a cause.
   E   infarction of bone shows on x-ray by increased radiolucency.

265. **In extracapsular fracture of the proximal femur**
   A   external rotation and shortening of the leg occurs.
   B   traction and bed-rest for three months is suitable treatment for the elderly patient.
   C   treatment by traction and rest is not acceptable in the treatment of young adults.
   D   simple nailing (such as the Smith-Petersen nail) is the most suitable treatment.
   E   avascular necrosis of the head is almost unknown.

266. **In an adult patient with a fracture of the shaft of the femur**
   A   no blood can be lost without obvious swelling.
   B   no blood can be lost without obvious bruising.
   C   two litres of blood can be lost without obvious swelling or bruising.
   D   there is no likelihood of death from haemorrhagic shock.
   E   fat embolism does not occur.

267. **The immediate management of condylar fractures of the femur includes**
   A   Kuntscher nailing.
   B   arthrodesis.
   C   skeletal traction.
   D   a plaster of Paris cylinder.
   E   a Milwaukee brace.

268. **A fracture of the patella can be classified as being**
   A   undisplaced transverse.
   B   vertical.
   C   osteochondral.
   D   a Salter type.
   E   a fatigue fracture.

269. **Fractures of the patella**
   A   can be caused by indirect violence.
   B   are stellate in appearance if caused by indirect violence.
   C   if stellate are treated by circumferential wiring.
   D   if transverse are best treated by patellectomy.
   E   are never vertical fractures.

270. **Treatment of a severe comminuted fracture of the patella includes**
   A   physiotherapy alone.
   B   insertion of a figure-of-eight tension band.
   C   patellectomy.
   D   inserting screws or wire.
   E   skin traction.

271. **In dislocation of the patella**
   A   the patella dislocates to the medial side of the knee.
   B   the knee becomes locked.
   C   the condition is predisposed to by an unusually high lateral femoral condyle.
   D   the condition is liable to recur spontaneously.
   E   patellectomy is the most suitable treatment.

272. **Features recognised as being associated with the diagnosis of ruptured anterior cruciate ligament include**
   A   minor swelling.
   B   little pain.
   C   haemarthrosis.
   D   dislocation of the patella.
   E   excessive posterior glide.

273. **Features in the knee recognised as being consistent with a torn medial meniscus include**
   A   swelling.
   B   excessive forward glide.
   C   locking.
   D   McMurray's sign.
   E   giving way.

274. **Examples of traction injuries include**
   A   fracture of the medial tibial tubercle.
   B   fracture of the medial epicondyle of the humerus.
   C   fracture of the medial malleolus of the tibia.
   D   mallet finger.
   E   stellate fracture of the patella.

275. **Fractures of the tibia and fibula**
    A   are often compound.
    B   are suitable for treatment by plaster after manipulative reduction in patients under 16 years.
    C   cannot be treated by skeletal traction.
    D   are most easily and safely treated by internal fixation with an intramedullary nail or plates and screws.
    E   can support weight without a plaster after eight weeks of immobilisation.

276. **In fractures involving the ankle joint**
    A   the stability of the tibiofibular mortice determines the outcome.
    B   if the mortice is disrupted it must be reconstructed.
    C   in a third-degree external rotation injury the talus is free to slide beneath, and possibly fracture, the posterior margin of the tibia.
    D   in an inversion (adduction) injury the medial malleolus may be sheared from the tibia.
    E   diastasis of the inferior tibiofibular joint is caused by a vertical compression injury.

277. **To deduce the mechanism of an ankle injury, the key is the radio-logical appearance of the fibular fracture, namely**
    A   low transverse = inversion injury usually.
    B   high in the shaft = eversion injury.
    C   spiral at the level of the inferior tibiofibular joint = internal rotation injury.
    D   high transverse = external rotation injury.
    E   low transverse = transverse shear.

278. **In fracture of the os calcis**
    A   the spine of the patient should be x-rayed.
    B   the bone is shattered like an eggshell.
    C   usually the subtalar joint is spared.
    D   the heel is inverted.
    E   skeletal traction is employed.

279. **Transmetatarsal dislocation is**
    A   associated with a march fracture of the metatarsals.
    B   synonymous with Lisfranc's dislocation.
    C   associated with ischaemia of the toes.
    D   part of neuropathic arthropathy.
    E   treated by open reduction.

Chapter 6

Diseases of bones and joints

280. In acute osteomyelitis
   A   the bone infarct is called a sequestrum.
   B   antibiotics will sterilise a sequestrum.
   C   ensheathing new bone is called an involucrum.
   D   if an involucrum should form it has to be removed totally before cure is possible.
   E   discharge through the involucrum is by means of holes known as cloacae.

281. Acute osteomyelitis
   A   can be fatal in children.
   B   is a haematogenous infection.
   C   begins in the epiphysis.
   D   begins under the periosteum.
   E   causes bone dysplasia.

282. In the management of acute osteomyelitis
   A   a single venepuncture for blood culture will always suffice to confirm the diagnosis.
   B   x-ray showing lifting of the periosteum is seen immediately.
   C   antibiotics should not be given until the results of culture and sensitivity are known.
   D   pus, if its presence is suspected clinically, should be drained by operation.
   E   operation should be carried out with the limb exsanguinated.

283. Chronic osteomyelitis
   A   causes continuous symptoms and signs over a period of months or years
   B   on x-ray may reveal a sequestrum.
   C   on x-ray may reveal a cavity.
   D   if a Brodie's abscess, reveals a band of sclerosis around a central lucent area on x-ray.
   E   nowadays is always cured by a long course of antibiotics.

284. Acute suppurative arthritis
  A can be caused by a penetrating wound.
  B can be caused by a compound fracture involving a joint.
  C can be due to blood-borne infection with the gonococcus.
  D causes dislocation.
  E inevitably results in ankylosis of the fibrous type.

285. The position of ease that joints take up in acute suppurative arthritis includes, the
  A shoulder – abducted.
  B elbow – extended and supinated.
  C hip – flexed, abducted and internally rotated.
  D knee – straight.
  E ankle – dorsiflexed.

286. The most suitable positions for ankylosis of a joint include, the
  A elbow if unilateral – 90° of flexion semi-pronated.
  B wrist – slightly dorsiflexed.
  C hip – 60° of flexion to allow sitting in a chair.
  D knee –30° of flexion to allow sitting in a chair.
  E ankle – at a right angle.

287. The diagnosis and management of tuberculous arthritis includes
  A waiting for a positive culture of the tubercle bacillus before treatment is started.
  B biopsy of lymph nodes.
  C incision to let out pus.
  D arthrotomy.
  E arthrodesis.

288. Pott's paraplegia is associated with
  A damage to the cord by a sequestrum.
  B the presence of tuberculous pus and angulation of the spine.
  C ischaemia of the anterior spinal arteries.
  D corda equina damage after a fall.
  E fracture dislocation of cervical vertebrae.

289. 'Melon seed' bodies are found in
  A the peritoneal cavity following pancreatitis.
  B a bunion.
  C a compound palmar ganglion.
  D the bladder in tuberculous cystitis.
  E the CSF.

290. With tuberculous infection of bones and joints
A the primary focus may be in the gastrointestinal tract.
B the condition is always due to the human strain of *Mycobacterium tuberculosis.*
C the disease starts in bone and not synovial membrane.
D a joint may dislocate following destruction of bone.
E bony ankylosis is the final outcome if treatment is satisfactory.

291. Benign tumours of bones and joints include
A osteoid osteoma.
B aneurysmal bone cyst.
C fibroma.
D Ewing's tumour.
E synovial sarcoma.

292. The malignant tumours of bone include the
A osteoclastoma.
B 'brown' tumour.
C chondrosarcoma.
D neuroblastoma.
E meningioma.

293. Features characteristic of osteosarcoma include
A pathological fracture.
B origination in the epiphyseal region.
C cellular pleomorphism.
D soap-bubble appearances on x-ray.
E ready radiosensitivity.

294. Features characteristic of osteoclastoma include
A pathological fracture.
B origin in the metaphyseal region.
C the display of 'sun ray' spicules on x-ray.
D predilection for the female sex.
E recurrence following local removal.

295. Ewing's tumour affecting the humerus
A is a metastasis from carcinoma of the thyroid.
B should be treated by immediate amputation.
C looks like a cut onion on x-ray.
D has a soap-bubble appearance on x-ray.
E displays sun-ray spicules on x-ray.

296. **A giant cell tumour of bone will show on x-ray**
   A   sun-ray spicules.
   B   Codman's triangle.
   C   a soap-bubble appearance.
   D   spotty calcification.
   E   onion layering.

297. **An ecchondroma**
   A   grows in the medulla of bone.
   B   grows on the surface of bone.
   C   is due to rickets.
   D   can undergo malignant change if the tumour is solitary.
   E   occurs in the phalanges.

298. **Paget's disease of bone**
   A   can affect any bone in the body.
   B   appears primarily as an osteosclerosis.
   C   causes deafness.
   D   produces bone that is stronger than normal bone.
   E   affects cancellous and cortical bone.

299. **The recognised consequences of Paget's disease of bone include**
   A   bone marrow suppression.
   B   left ventricular failure.
   C   meningioma.
   D   festinant gait.
   E   paraplegia.

300. **Senile osteoporosis**
   A   can only be detected radiologically when about 40% of the skeleton has been lost.
   B   is manifest on x-ray of the spine as a 'fish head' appearance of the vertebral bodies.
   C   causes much bone pain.
   D   causes delayed healing if a fracture occurs.
   E   is, through progressive fatigue, a likely cause of fracture of the neck of the femur.

301. **Osteomalacia**
   A   is rickets in the adult skeleton.
   B   is due to deficient absorption of vitamin A.
   C   is associated with blind loop syndrome.
   D   is consistent with a raised serum alkaline phosphatase.
   E   can be brought about by renal tubular acidosis.

302. **Pathological changes in osteoarthritis include**
   A   fibrillation.
   B   ulceration.
   C   pannus formation.
   D   sclerosis.
   E   cyst formation.

303. **Secondary osteoarthritis due to articular cartilage damage is associated with**
   A   Paget's disease.
   B   slipped femoral epiphysis.
   C   gonococcal arthritis.
   D   chondrocalcinosis.
   E   osteomalacia.

304. **Osteoarthritis**
   A   causes muscle spasm.
   B   is primarily due to abrasion caused by a breakdown in joint lubrication.
   C   is manifested in the first place by fibrillation of articular cartilage.
   D   causes fibrosis of the capsule of a joint.
   E   causes the appearance of bone 'cysts' in cancellous bone adjacent to a joint.

305. **The clinical features that are associated with osteoarthritis of the hip include**
   A   pain on walking but not at night.
   B   muscle spasm.
   C   the joint being held in the position of ease which is functionally useless.
   D   apparent shortening.
   E   telescopic movement.

306. **Characteristic radiological appearances of osteoarthritis include**
   A   widening of the joint space.
   B   new bone formation.
   C   subchondral sclerosis.
   D   subluxation.
   E   Codman's triangle.

307. **Pathological changes in rheumatoid arthritis of the knee include**
   A   synovial infiltration with plasma cells.
   B   effusion.
   C   synovial pannus.
   D   destruction of the cruciate ligaments.
   E   osteosclerosis.

308. **Characteristic features of rheumatoid arthritis include**
   A   appearance in childhood.
   B   affects men more than women.
   C   mild fever.
   D   persistently unremitting pain and stiffness.
   E   muscle wasting.

309. **Surgery in relation to the pathology of osteoarthritis includes**
   A   osteotomy.
   B   arthrodesis.
   C   synovectomy.
   D   replacement arthroplasty.
   E   sympathectomy.

310. **Operations favoured for rheumatoid arthritis include**
   A   osteotomy.
   B   replacement arthroplasty.
   C   synovectomy.
   D   neurectomy.
   E   excision arthroplasty.

311. **Ankylosing spondylitis**
   A   affects the small distal joints in the extremities first.
   B   is more common in women than in men.
   C   is associated with pulmonary fibrosis.
   D   characteristically displays tissue antigen HLA-B27.
   E   is associated with aortic valve disease.

312. **Ankylosing spondylitis**
   A   can be regarded as a variant of rheumatoid arthritis.
   B   is a process of calcification and ossification of cartilage.
   C   is associated with spondylolisthesis.
   D   can be partly diagnosed by tissue typing.
   E   tends to begin in the sacroiliac joints.

313. **Congenital dislocation of the hip is**
   A   bilateral.
   B   associated with a hereditary predisposition to joint laxity.
   C   part of the Ehlers-Danlos syndrome.
   D   commoner in the male than in the female.
   E   associated with breech presentation.

314. **A positive Trendelenburg's sign**
   A   is present when the pelvis rises on the unsupported side on walking.
   B   occurs with paralysis of hip adductors.
   C   occurs with coxa vara.
   D   on both sides can make the gait appear normal.
   E   on one side causes a lurching gait downwards towards the unsupported side.

315. **If an unstable hip is detected at birth the management policy is to**
   A   do nothing and re-examine every six months as only a minority of hips develop into a persistent dislocation.
   B   use a splint to keep the hip joint in 45° flexion and adduction.
   C   use a splint to keep the hip joint in 90° flexion and abduction.
   D   advise operative stabilisation.
   E   use a Thomas' thigh splint.

316. **In the case of unilateral congenital dislocation of the hip in children aged between six months and seven years**
   A   reduction should be effected and maintained.
   B   the older the child the more difficult the reduction becomes.
   C   maintenance of reduction may be difficult because the acetabulum is abnormally shallow and vertical.
   D   open reduction should always be performed.
   E   the results of treatment are worse than the disease itself.

317. **Coxa vara is associated with**
   A   an increase in angle between the femoral neck and the femoral shaft.
   B   femoral dysplasia.
   C   defective endochondral ossification of the head of the femur.
   D   fractured neck of femur.
   E   rickets.

318. **Club foot is**
   A   more common in girls than in boys.
   B   associated with CDH.
   C   associated with Freeman-Sheldon syndrome.
   D   most commonly of the equinovalgus variety.
   E   characteristically associated with a breech presentation.

319. **Recognised features of club foot include**
   A   erosion of the os calcis.
   B   adduction of the bones of the forefoot.
   C   a small os calcis.
   D   calf muscle wasting.
   E   scleroderma.

320. **In a neonate with club foot**
   A   the foot can be dorsiflexed until the dorsum touches the shin.
   B   arthrogryphosis can be present.
   C   x-ray is necessary for diagnosis.
   D   the mother can be taught manipulation therapy if the deformity is slight.
   E   a Denis Browne splint can be used.

321. **The condition known as osteogenesis imperfecta is**
   A   a recognised consequence of the mother taking thalidomide.
   B   inherited.
   C   associated with laxity of ligaments.
   D   likely if Wormian bones are present.
   E   eventually resolved as osteopetrosis.

322. **Diaphyseal aclasia**
   A   is more common in females than males.
   B   is an autosomal dominant inherited condition.
   C   can interfere with muscle function.
   D   ceases activity at maturity.
   E   does not become malignant.

323. **Idiopathic scoliosis is a**
   A   lateral curvature of the spine.
   B   rotation of the spine.
   C   lateral curvature with rotation of the spine.
   D   flexion deformity of the spine.
   E   congenital disease with hemivertebrae.

324. **Congenital torticollis**
  A is a true congenital abnormality.
  B involves infarcted muscles.
  C exhibits a swelling called a potato tumour.
  D causes facial asymmetry.
  E is treated by division of the accessory nerve.

325. **The types of scoliosis include the**
  A congenital.
  B paralytic.
  C postural.
  D pulmonary.
  E gastro-oesophageal.

326. **Recognised current procedures in the management of scoliosis include**
  A repeated comparable A-P x-rays of the spine.
  B the use of the Milwaukee brace.
  C the use of plaster casts.
  D insertion of rods and hooks.
  E insertion of Rush nails.

327. **A slipped femoral epiphysis**
  A is due to infarction of the epiphysis.
  B occurs in overweight multipara.
  C occurs in overweight boys aged between 10 and 18 years.
  D affects overweight girls aged between four and eight years.
  E follows surgery.

328. **Factors predisposing to slipped femoral epiphysis include**
  A high normal loads.
  B rickets.
  C 'hypogonadal' children.
  D an epiphyseal plate not disposed at right angles to the line of action of the resultant force applied to it.
  E previous poliomyelitis.

329. **Features associated with chronic slipped epiphysis include**
  A knock knee.
  B pain in the knee.
  C in-toeing.
  D apparent shortening.
  E isolated limitation of external rotation and abduction.

330. **The essential examination of the hip in order to clinch the diagnosis of chronic slipped femoral epiphysis is**
   A   measuring for shortening of the leg.
   B   palpation of the femoral head.
   C   A-P plain x-ray view of the hip.
   D   lateral x-ray view of the hip.
   E   the Trendelenburg test.

331. **The management of acute slipped epiphysis in a young adult includes**
   A   Denis Browne splints.
   B   a Milwaukee brace.
   C   osteoclasis.
   D   internal fixation with three threaded pins.
   E   diet.

332. **Traction injuries of the epiphyses include**
   A   Sever's disease.
   B   Osgood Schlatter's disease.
   C   Kienbock's disease.
   D   Scheuermann's disease.
   E   Freiberg's disease.

333. **In Perthe's disease of the head of the femur**
   A   girls are more commonly affected than boys.
   B   the condition presents with a limp.
   C   the younger the child the worse the prognosis.
   D   if the femoral head becomes deformed osteoarthritis can occur in adult life.
   E   the most effective way of reducing the chances of a deformed head of femur is to confine the child to bed for two to three years.

334. **The radiological features associated with Perthe's disease include**
   A   an enlarged ossific nucleus.
   B   an enlarged joint space.
   C   epiphyseal fragmentation.
   D   lateral subluxation.
   E   a horizontal growth plate.

335. The management of Perthe's disease includes
  A   no treatment.
  B   broomstick plasters.
  C   compression nail plating.
  D   femoral osteotomy.
  E   innominate osteotomy.

336. There is a recognised association between
  A   rickets and knock knee.
  B   Blount's disease and bow leg.
  C   in-toeing and knock knee.
  D   slipped femoral epiphysis and bow leg.
  E   osteochondritis and knock knee.

Chapter 7

Disorders of muscles, tendons and ligaments
Sports-related injuries
The hand
The foot

337. **Tennis elbow is**
   A also known as medial epicondylitis.
   B characteristically associated with tenderness of the attachment of the extensor muscles of the forearm.
   C associated with the presence of bone chips.
   D treated by rest.
   E associated with olecranon bursitis.

338. **There is a recognised association between**
   A tennis elbow and acute suppurative tenosynovitis.
   B tenosynovitis and melon-seed bodies.
   C melon-seed bodies and peritoneal mice.
   D peritoneal mice and breast mice.
   E breast mice and fibroadenoma.

339. **Muscles at risk from exercise injury include**
   A those that span two joints.
   B those that work eccentrically.
   C those that contain a high proportion of type 2 fibres.
   D the rectus femoris.
   E the pectoralis major.

340. **Intermuscular bleeding caused by a direct blow**
   A causes more pain than intramuscular bleeding.
   B causes more inhibition of movement than intramuscular bleeding.
   C results in distant bruising according to the force of gravity.
   D is very likely to result in myositis ossificans.
   E is likely to result in cyst formation.

341. **Supraspinatus tendon lesions are associated with**
   A tendon ischaemia.
   B acutely painful calcific tendonitis.
   C inability to initiate adduction of the shoulder.
   D degeneration of the tendon.
   E inevitable frozen shoulder.

342. **Patella tendonosis**
   A   is associated with myxoid degeneration.
   B   occurs in sprinters.
   C   occurs predominantly in females.
   D   causes pain on sitting.
   E   should be managed by patellectomy.

343. **A patient with stenosing tenovaginitis**
   A   is likely to have a Dupuytren's contracture.
   B   has carpal tunnel syndrome.
   C   may suffer from trigger finger.
   D   has thickening of tendon sheaths to the fingers and thumb.
   E   is likely to have iritis.

344. **A trigger finger is**
   A   an inflamed index finger.
   B   an atrophic index finger in a median nerve palsy.
   C   due to stenosing tenovaginitis affecting one of the flexor tendons in the palm.
   D   an essential feature of the carpal tunnel syndrome.
   E   a component of syndactyly.

345. **A ganglion**
   A   is due to neurofibromatosis.
   B   can be painless.
   C   may be due to leakage of synovial fluid through the capsule of a joint.
   D   is best excised under a local anaesthetic.
   E   if untreated becomes a 'compound palmar ganglion'.

346. **The causes of bursitis are recognised to include**
   A   trauma.
   B   pyogenic infection.
   C   gonorrhoea.
   D   syphilis.
   E   tuberculosis.

347. **A Baker's cyst is**
   A   an implantation dermoid cyst occurring in the palms of those who work in a bakery.
   B   a synovial cyst of the wrists of those who knead bread.
   C   a prepatellar bursa.
   D   a synovial cyst of the ankle.
   E   a synovial cyst of the popliteal fossa.

348. **An adventitious bursa is**
    A   an anatomical bursa overlying any joint.
    B   a type of degeneration of the adventitia of the popliteal artery.
    C   an acquired bursa generated from connective tissue.
    D   a pseudocyst in the lesser sac (omental bursa).
    E   an infected knee.

349. **The principles to be followed in the treatment of infections of the hand include**
    A   rest.
    B   elevation of the limb.
    C   accurate localisation of pain.
    D   evacuation of pus.
    E   antibiotic therapy.

350. **Anaesthesia for operations on the fingers include the use of**
    A   simple gas and oxygen.
    B   2% lignocaine.
    C   muscle relaxants.
    D   brachial plexus block.
    E   epidural anaesthesia.

351. **The treatment of acute paronychia includes**
    A   flucloxacillin.
    B   operative gentle stripping of eponychium to release pus.
    C   always avulsion of the nail.
    D   excision of loose eponychium.
    E   griseofulvin.

352. **Features likely to be present in acute terminal pulp-space infection include**
    A   pain on elevation of the hand.
    B   throbbing pain.
    C   osteomyelitis of the whole terminal phalanx.
    D   interference with sleep.
    E   lymphangitis.

353. **Concerning the surgery of a pulp infection of the finger**
    A   only when pus is present should the abscess be uncapped.
    B   a long incision is necessary in the long axis of the pulp.
    C   a collar stud abscess may be present.
    D   a slough must be looked for and carefully excised.
    E   the periosteum of the terminal phalanx should be incised.

354. If a patient has a web space infection

A there is considerable oedema of the back of the hand.

B the patient is kept under observation being given a sling and asked to attend the clinic every day.

C antibiotics are withheld until pus has formed.

D the infection fortunately remains localised to that web space.

E the space is approached surgically through a transverse incision.

355. With a deep palmar abscess

A the patient is usually a manual worker.

B there is intense throbbing pain in the palm of the hand.

C a 'frog hand' may appear.

D extension of the I-P joints characteristically is exquisitely painful.

E trimming back incised palmar skin and fascia is necessary to prevent premature healing.

356. Kanavel's sign is

A swelling above the flexor retinaculum.

B flexion of the thumb when the radial bursa is infected.

C flexion of the fingers in a compound palmar ganglion.

D tenderness over an infected ulnar bursa between the transverse palmar creases.

E oedema of the dorsum of the hand.

357. The space of Parona is

A in the wrist between the deep flexor tendons and the pronator quadratus.

B above the patella between the quadriceps muscle and the femur.

C beneath the tendon of the iliopsoas.

D between the Achilles' tendon and the posterior aspect of the tibia.

E in the web space of the palm.

358. In acute suppurative tenosynovitis

A septicaemia can occur.

B the organism may be *Streptococcus pyogenes*.

C the whole finger is swollen.

D the finger is flexed.

E there is exquisite pain on passive extension.

359. In the management of hand injuries

A primary repair of nerves and tendons is always advisable in any type of hand injury.

B the hand should be exsanguinated for the operation.

C an untidy wound should be left open to granulate and heal by second intention.

D immediately after operation the hand should be nursed flat.

E postoperatively early movement is essential to prevent stiffness.

360. With tendon and nerve injuries in the hand

A all types of division are best sutured immediately.

B extensor tendon suture gives poor results.

C in the palm the suture of both sublimis and profundus tendons can be carried out at the same operation.

D the digital sheath should be repaired if possible.

E primary suture is preferable for digital nerve surgery.

361. The maximum safe time that a tourniquet may be left on for the purpose of obtaining a bloodless field in hand surgery is (should not exceed)

A 30 minutes.

B 45 minutes.

C one hour.

D one hour 30 minutes.

E two hours.

362. A Dupuytren's contracture

A is a contraction of flexor tendons.

B commonly involves the finger.

C can be present in the foot.

D is treated by tendon-lengthening procedures.

E may well be seen in people with epilepsy, cirrhosis of the liver or Peyronie's disease.

363. There is a recognised association between carpal tunnel syndrome and

A Dupuytren's contracture.

B rheumatoid arthritis.

C pregnancy.

D compound palmar ganglion.

E Sudeck's atrophy.

364. There is a recognised association between

A the cause of ingrowing toenail and subungual exostosis.

B Madura foot and leprosy.

C flat foot and infants.

D pes cavus and Friedreich's ataxia

E hallux valgus and hammer toe.

365. The treatments appropriate to the named lesions includes

A wedge resection and precise phenolisation of the nail matrix for ingrowing toenail.

B removal of the terminal phalanx for onychogryphosis.

C excision of an infected adventitious bursa of the foot.

D wide spectrum antibiotics and dapsone for Madura foot.

E medial incision of the sole of the foot for the drainage of pus.

366. Infection of the heel space

A is always due to puncture by a nail or a needle.

B can have a collar stud extension into a deeper plane.

C is associated with oedema of the ankle.

D spreads among the fibrous septa, which require division on treatment.

E is commonly by *Pseudomonas aeruginosa*.

367. 'Idiopathic' adult flat foot is primarily due to

A collapse of the lateral longitudinal arch.

B overstretched plantar ligaments.

C collapse of the medial longitudinal arch.

D a congenital bar of bone between the talus and the navicular bone.

E plantar fasciitis.

368. In pes cavus

A the instep is high with flattening and splaying of the toes.

B the deformity seems to be caused by weakness of the intrinsic muscles of the foot.

C another factor causing the deformity is the presence of a Dupuytren's contracture of the plantar fascia.

D in childhood the foot is painful and the contracted plantar fascia is tender.

E Friedreich's ataxia should be excluded.

369. Features associated with hallux valgus include

  A   an overriding of the second toe by the first.
  B   an underriding of the second toe by the first.
  C   rheumatoid arthritis of the first metatarsophalangeal joint.
  D   an inflamed adventitious bursa.
  E   an exostosis on the lateral side of the head of the first metatarsal.

370. A bunion is

  A   an exostosis of the base of the first metatarsal.
  B   a type of sesamoid bone.
  C   an inflamed adventitious bursa beside the head of the first metatarsal.
  D   an exostosis of the head of the first metatarsal.
  E   a verucca.

371. There is a recognised association between

  A   hallux rigidus and osteochondritis dissecans.
  B   hammer toes and callosities.
  C   claw toes and pes cavus.
  D   Madura mycosis and march fracture.
  E   plantar fasciitis and spastic flat foot.

Chapter 8

Neurological disorders

372. In the management of patients with muscular paralysis acceptable measures include
A   converting a spastic paralysis into a flaccid paralysis.
B   allowing flexors and adductors to overcome extensors.
C   the use of orthotics.
D   tendon lengthening in spastic paralysis.
E   arthrodesis.

373. Acceptable tendon transfers in cases of muscular paralysis include
A   transferring part of pectoralis major to the inferior angle of the scapula for winging of the scapula.
B   the transfer of the triceps into the distal biceps tendon for paralysis of the musculocutaneous nerve.
C   transferring pronator teres into the extensor carpi ulnaris for radial nerve palsy.
D   transferring brachioradialis into the flexor pollicis longus for medial nerve lesions.
E   the transfer of the tibialis anterior into the tibialis posterior for lateral popliteal lesions.

374. Acceptable treatments in cerebral palsy include
A   adductor tenotomy for scissors gait.
B   hamstring tenotomy for knee extension deformity.
C   full Achilles' tenotomy for equinus deformity.
D   flexor slide for finger flexion deformity.
E   strengthening abductors and extensors, releasing thenar muscles and lengthening flexor pollicis longus for thumb adduction deformity.

375. Friedreich's ataxia
A   is an X-linked recessive condition.
B   affects part of the cerebellum.
C   is associated with patchy demyelination.
D   presents at maturity.
E   causes bilateral pes cavus.

376. **Poliomyelitis is recognised to be associated with**
   A   pes calcaneus due to paralysis of the tibialis anterior.
   B   dislocation of the hip.
   C   Raynaud's phenomenon.
   D   neuropathic joints.
   E   scoliosis.

377. **Unstable injuries of the spine include**
   A   fractured transverse process.
   B   crush fracture of the body, dorsal spine.
   C   fracture dislocation dorsilumbar junction.
   D   fractured odontoid.
   E   burst fracture.

378. **In a patient with spinal concussion**
   A   a spastic paralysis occurs below the site of the lesion.
   B   there is abolition of reflex activity below the lesion.
   C   joint position sense is lost.
   D   pain and temperature sense is lost.
   E   if there is no partial or complete cord injury, power and sensation should take 7–10 days to return.

379. **Below the level of the lesion in spinal concussion the characteristic features include**
   A   a flaccid paralysis.
   B   retention of urine.
   C   loss of reflexes.
   D   loss of sensation.
   E   Froin's syndrome.

380. **The types of presentation of incomplete spinal cord injury include**
   A   that of the anterior cord associated with loss of joint position sense and vibration.
   B   that of the posterior cord associated with loss of pain and temperature sense.
   C   Brown-Séquard's syndrome of ipsilateral weakness and contralateral loss of pain and temperature sensation.
   D   the central lesion with incomplete tetraparesis.
   E   the central lesion with lower limbs characteristically more severely affected than the upper.

381. Traumatic intraspinal haemorrhage due to spinal trauma is manifested as
A haematomyelia defined as extradural haemorrhage.
B haematorrachis defined as haemorrhage within the cord.
C extradural haemorrhage causing (Thorburn's) gravitational paraplegia.
D immediate paralysis due to haematomyelia.
E delayed signs, e.g. muscle wasting.

382. The cause of death after a traumatic transection of the cord includes
A cerebral abscess.
B aerocele.
C pyelonephritis.
D bedsores.
E surgical emphysema.

383. In a fifth cervical complete cord lesion, paralysis occurs in
A the arms.
B the chest.
C the diaphragm.
D the legs.
E the platysma.

384. In the management of a patient with a spinal cord injury
A the patient should be turned every six hours.
B plaster immobilisation increases the risk of pressure sores.
C meteorism should be allowed to occur.
D passive movements of the limbs are necessary.
E operations such as plating are indicated to relieve existing damage to the cord.

385. After a collision a motorcyclist is thrown into the air and falls to sustain a thoracolumbar fracture dislocation which can feature
A abrasions over the scapula.
B a boggy haematoma over the area.
C a palpable gap between the spinal processes.
D on x-ray a burst fracture.
E on x-ray a horizontal slice fracture.

386. **Recognised features of spina bifida include**
  A   foot drop.
  B   enuresis.
  C   a lipoma.
  D   a hairy patch.
  E   a meningocele.

387. **Open neural tube defects**
  A   are congenital lesions, not familial.
  B   are likely to occur in subsequent pregnancies.
  C   can all be picked up during pregnancy by maternal serum screening and amniocentesis.
  D   can be associated with Budd-Chiari syndrome.
  E   are associated with normal intelligence.

388. **If a child is born with myelocele**
  A   gross talipes is obvious.
  B   meningitis is likely to occur.
  C   the swelling contains only cerebrospinal fluid.
  D   an elliptical raw surface is seen.
  E   operation should be delayed for three months.

389. **In relation to tumours of the vertebral column**
  A   secondary deposits far outweigh primary tumours.
  B   of the secondary deposits, the majority originate from a primary bronchial carcinoma.
  C   a chordoma usually originates in the thoracic spine.
  D   multiple myelomas masquerade as osteoporosis.
  E   x-ray will show prostate secondaries as characteristically being osteolytic.

390. **With tumours of the spinal canal**
  A   dumb-bell tumours are extradural neurofibromas.
  B   neurofibromas may cause erosion of an intervertebral foramen.
  C   intradural tumours can be meningiomas.
  D   approximately 50% of intramedullary tumours are gliomas.
  E   the commonest extradural tumour is the spinal metastasis.

391. **In the diagnosis of spinal cord tumours**
    A   lumbar puncture is helpful.
    B   plain x-ray can show scalloping of the posterior margins of the vertebral bodies.
    C   plain x-ray can show enlarged intervertebral foramina.
    D   MRI can differentiate between solid and cystic tumours.
    E   gadolinium assists in identifying the nature of the tumour.

392. **Intramedullary tumours of the cord cause**
    A   early prominent root pain.
    B   dissociated sensory loss.
    C   early bladder symptoms.
    D   early spasticity.
    E   a belt of local sensory loss.

393. **Clinical features relating to lumbosacral disc compression involving the fourth lumbar root include**
    A   sensory loss in the groin.
    B   weak gastrocnemius.
    C   weak quadriceps.
    D   absent ankle jerk.
    E   diminished knee jerk.

394. **A lateral protrusion of a C6 disc produces**
    A   pain in the tip of the shoulder.
    B   sensory loss of the lateral border of the upper arm.
    C   weakness of the trapezius.
    D   a diminished triceps jerk.
    E   a diminished supinator jerk.

395. **Trigeminal neuralgia**
    A   is known as *tic douloureux*.
    B   is pain mainly in the first division of the fifth nerve.
    C   is helped by rubbing the part of the face affected.
    D   is a constant pain.
    E   has recognised association with migraine.

396. **The facial nerve**
    A   is an entirely motor nerve.
    B   gives a branch to the stapedius muscle.
    C   enters the neck through the stylomastoid foramen.
    D   lies deep to the styloid process.
    E   communicates with the auriculotemporal nerve.

397. A seventh nerve palsy

A   if due to an infranuclear lesion involves only the lower half of the face.

B   can be caused by middle ear disease.

C   is not always a Bell's palsy.

D   is an indication of malignancy when associated with a parotid tumour.

E   causes corneal ulceration.

398. The chorda tympani nerve

A   is a branch of the acoustic nerve.

B   passes forward between the fibrous and mucous layers of the tympanic membrane.

C   joins the lingual nerve.

D   fibres pass through the submandibular ganglion.

E   if severed on the excision of the submandibular salivary gland will result in loss of taste from the posterior third of the tongue.

399. The hypoglossal nerve in the neck

A   emerges between the internal carotid artery and the internal jugular vein.

B   loops round the upper sternomastoid branch of the occipital artery.

C   superficially crosses the tendon of the digastric and stylohyoid muscles.

D   is identifiable on the hyoglossus as it is accompanied by veins.

E   if severed on excision of the submandibular salivary gland causes deviation of the tongue to the opposite side on protrusion.

400. Neuropraxia characteristically is

A   intrathecal rupture of the nerve fibres within an intact sheath.

B   partial or complete division of nerve sheath and fibres.

C   physiological paralysis of the intact nerve fibres.

D   followed by degeneration of axons.

E   followed by complete recovery.

401. **In recovery from axonotmesis**
- **A** Wallerian degeneration has occurred in the distal portion of the broken axons leaving an empty tubule.
- **B** the Nissl granules reform.
- **C** the proliferating axons grow through the block caused by intraneural fibrosis.
- **D** the down-growing axons proceed immediately at the rate of 3 mm/day.
- **E** on arrival at the end-organs there is a delay of about three weeks before these end-organs are activated.

402. **In the repair of neurotmesis**
- **A** extensive mobilisation of nerve ends is preferable to inserting a graft.
- **B** bulging nerve bundles must be present in the ends before suture.
- **C** epineurium must be completely joined.
- **D** a healthy bed is essential.
- **E** frozen muscle grafts up to 4 cm can be used instead of nerve grafts.

403. **Nerve suture**
- **A** gives better results in adults than in children.
- **B** of proximal nerves give better results than suture of distal nerves.
- **C** of the motor nerves to the small muscles of the hand do well.
- **D** of motor nerves can lead to algodystrophy.
- **E** performed within 10 days of injury yields the best results.

404. **An upper brachial plexus lesion (Erb-Duchenne)**
- **A** only affects infants after a difficult labour.
- **B** affects the fifth dorsal nerve.
- **C** causes the arm to hang by the side with the forearm pronated.
- **D** involving the fifth nerve gives rise to an area of anaesthesia over the outer side of the arm.
- **E** can be treated by ankylosis.

405. **Avulsion of the first dorsal nerve root**
- **A** occurs in the case of a falling person clutching at an object and hyperabducting the arm.
- **B** causes paralysis of the intrinsic muscles of the hand.
- **C** causes anaesthesia in the anatomical snuff-box.
- **D** is likely to cause a Horner's syndrome.
- **E** can be the cause of some spasticity of the leg on the same side.

406. A Klumpke paralysis
  A   is a lower brachial plexus lesion.
  B   causes wasting of the thenar muscles only.
  C   causes sensory loss along the inner side of the forearm.
  D   causes sensory loss of the inner three-and-a-half fingers.
  E   is congenital.

407. If the circumflex (axillary nerve) is cut
  A   the deltoid muscle is paralysed.
  B   the triceps is paralysed,
  C   the teres minor is paralysed.
  D   there is a patch of anaesthesia in the anatomical snuff-box.
  E   the pectoralis minor muscle is paralysed.

408. Severance of the long nerve of Bell (the external respiratory nerve) causes
  A   paralysis of the serratus anterior.
  B   paralysis of the subscapularis.
  C   winging of the scapula.
  D   deficiency of the 'lunge' as in boxing or fencing.
  E   difficulty in raising the arm above a right angle from a position in front of the body.

409. Severance of the radial nerve in the axilla causes
  A   paralysis of the deltoid.
  B   inability to extend the elbow.
  C   complete inability to extend the fingers with the hand supported.
  D   inability to supinate the forearm.
  E   anaesthesia over the dorsum of the forearm.

410. A 'Saturday night' palsy is
  A   temporary lower limb paralysis due to alcoholic intoxication.
  B   acute retention of urine.
  C   due to injury to the radial nerve in the radial groove.
  D   a temporary squint.
  E   synonymous with carpal tunnel syndrome.

411. Severance of the radial nerve at the wrist results in
  A   *main en griffe*.
  B   wasting of the thenar eminence.
  C   wrist drop.
  D   trophic ulcer of the index finger.
  E   anaesthesia in the anatomical snuff-box.

412. **Severance of the median nerve at the elbow causes**
   A   paralysis of all the flexors of the fingers.
   B   fixed flexion of the terminal phalanx of the thumb.
   C   wasting of the hypothenar muscles.
   D   trophic changes in the index finger.
   E   loss of sensation at first over the thumb and radial two-and-a-half fingers.

413. **Ulnar nerve entrapment characteristically**
   A   is recognised in writers.
   B   is related to pressure on the ulnar nerve at the base of the hypothenar eminence.
   C   complicates Colles' fracture.
   D   results from an increased carrying angle after elbow fractures.
   E   presents early with pain.

414. **Severance of the ulnar nerve at the wrist causes**
   A   loss of sensation on the anterior and posterior aspects of the inner one-and-a half fingers.
   B   inability to flex the terminal phalanx of the little finger.
   C   flexion of the little finger at the metacarpophalangeal joint.
   D   inability to abduct or adduct the fingers.
   E   a positive Froment's sign.

415. **Complete severance of the lateral popliteal nerve**
   A   may be due to an injury to the upper end of the fibula.
   B   may be due to an operation for multiple ligation of varicose veins.
   C   causes a talipes equinovarus.
   D   causes anaesthesia of the outer sides of the fourth and fifth toes.
   E   causes anaesthesia of the front of the ligamentum patellae.

416. **Severance of the sciatic nerve high up causes**
   A   footdrop.
   B   complete inability to flex the knee.
   C   complete stocking anaesthesia.
   D   trophic ulcers.
   E   meralgia paraesthetica.

417. Causalgia

    A   tends to follow complete nerve injury.

    B   can be associated with a lateral neuroma.

    C   has physical signs produced by a histamine-like substance.

    D   can be relieved by paravertebral block.

    E   is associated with cold.

418. Of the swellings of the scalp and lumps on the head

    A   Cock's peculiar tumour is associated with oedema from underlying osteomyelitis of the skull.

    B   subaponeurotic bleeding in infants can cause decompensated hypovolaemia.

    C   an external angular dermoid can have an intracranial component.

    D   a midline swelling always requires imaging.

    E   an ivory osteoma is a type of diaphyseal aclasis.

419. Malignant growth involving the vault of the skull include

    A   osteitis fibrosa cystica.

    B   osteoclastoma.

    C   myeloid epulis.

    D   adamantinoma.

    E   nephroblastoma.

420. In relation to the types of cerebral injury, in

    A   concussion the pulse is full and bounding.

    B   concussion there is organic structural damage.

    C   cerebral contusion there is organic damage to nerve cells and axons.

    D   cerebral contusion the muscles are spastic.

    E   cerebral laceration damage to the tip of the temporal lobe causes traumatic anosmia.

421. The indications for admission of a patient following head injury include

    A   crime.

    B   absence of responsible relatives or friends.

    C   haemophilia.

    D   alcohol intoxication.

    E   the presence of focal neurological signs.

422. **The management of an unconscious patient with a head injury includes**
A   the patient being nursed in a darkened room.
B   an x-ray of the skull.
C   the patient being nursed strictly in the supine position.
D   immediate tracheostomy.
E   using a coma scale.

423. **In head injuries substances to be avoided in therapy include**
A   frusemide.
B   mannitol.
C   sulphonamides.
D   dicoumarol.
E   dexamethasone.

424. **The management of an unconscious patient includes such measures as**
A   constant traction on the tongue with a towel clip.
B   controlled ventilation.
C   anticonvulsants.
D   sedatives *per se*.
E   nursing in the supine position.

425. **In extradural haemorrhage**
A   the dura becomes forcibly detached from the skull at the site of injury.
B   a lucid interval between concussion and cerebral compression is always present.
C   constriction of the pupil on the affected side can always be observed in the course of making a diagnosis.
D   coning is unlikely to occur.
E   the patient must be operated upon on the next operating list.

426. **Subdural haemorrhage is**
A   six times less common than extradural haemorrhage.
B   particularly common in young people.
C   a cause of slowing of cerebration which comes and goes.
D   a cause of a midbrain pressure cone.
E   characterised by papilloedema.

427. **Regarding the management of scalp and skull injuries**
   A   on examination of the wound in the accident-receiving room a finger should be inserted to detect the presence of a compound fracture and brain damage.
   B   for a closed depressed fracture immediate operation is indicated.
   C   all scalp wounds should be explored adequately.
   D   a general anaesthetic is always necessary.
   E   any loose pieces of fractured skull should be removed and discarded as they will encourage infection.

428. **In a patient with an anterior fossa fracture**
   A   proptosis can occur.
   B   any subconjunctival haemorrhage is wedge-shaped with the apex at the back.
   C   the injury characteristically includes a tear of the tentorium.
   D   an aerocele can form.
   E   the optic nerve is frequently torn.

429. **The management of a patient with a fractured base of skull includes**
   A   propping up the patient to lower pressure and diminish the escape of cerebrospinal fluid.
   B   incising the suboccipital region if bruising and a boggy swelling in the nape of the neck or below the mastoid process suggest a posterior fossa fracture.
   C   withholding antibiotics until signs of infection are present.
   D   finding out if an aerocele is present.
   E   early repair of a dural gap.

430. **The late effects of a head injury include**
   A   symptomatic fits in the first 24 hours that recur after bruising has subsided.
   B   the Panda sign.
   C   headache which is not cerebral but is spinal in origin.
   D   Jacksonian epilepsy.
   E   idiopathic epileptic fits.

431. **The value of a CT scan in craniocerebral injury is to use it to**
   A   differentiate between brain swelling and a scalp swelling.
   B   differentiate between contusion and compression haematoma.
   C   demonstrate the thickness of an intracranial haematoma.
   D   monitor cerebral oedema.
   E   negate the need for a plain x-ray of the skull.

432. In cone formation

A   the temporal lobe may be forced downwards into the tentorial opening.

B   the cerebellar vermis may be pushed upwards into the tentorial opening.

C   the cerebellar tonsils may be forced downwards into the foramen magnum.

D   unilateral pupillary dilation is an urgent sign.

E   lumbar puncture to drain CSF relieves the condition.

433. The procedure for a first exploratory burr hole in a head injury which is compound includes

A   using an ethanol-based skin preparation.

B   making a horizontal incision immediately above the zygoma.

C   stripping the periosteum.

D   using a Hudson's brace firstly with a burr and then completing with a perforator.

E   enlarging the hole if necessary with bone rongeurs.

434. The clinical features of chronic subdural haematoma include

A   always a preceding loss of consciousness.

B   an extensor plantar response.

C   slowness of response to questions.

D   stupor which may come and go.

E   pupillary changes.

435. Regarding the diagnosis of intracerebral abscess

A   there can be evidence of past middle ear infection.

B   persistent pyrexia is frequently absent.

C   as the abscess enlarges the pulse rate may become slower.

D   leucocytosis does not occur because of the blood-brain barrier.

E   a lumbar puncture should not be performed as it can precipitate rupture of the abscess.

436. The types of glioma of the brain include

A   medulloblastoma.

B   acoustic neuroma.

C   astrocytoma.

D   meningioma.

E   oligodendroglioma.

437. Characteristics of meningiomas include
  A   endothelioma formation.
  B   flat features.
  C   reactive hyperostosis.
  D   the fact that about 18% of intracranial tumours are meningiomas.
  E   an origin in the arachnoid.

438. Craniopharyngiomas
  A   are calcified in 50% of cases.
  B   are removable.
  C   form large masses.
  D   have cystic cavities.
  E   cause hydrocephalus.

439. Regarding the presentation and diagnosis of cerebral tumour
  A   neurological examination usually indicates the type of tumour.
  B   a high ESR is strongly suggestive of secondary tumour.
  C   primary cerebral tumour is more common than metastatic carcinoma.
  D   30% of bronchial carcinomas present with cerebral symptoms before any chest symptoms have occurred.
  E   erosion of the posterior clinoid processes suggests that removal of the tumour may be possible.

440. The management of patients with cerebral tumours includes
  A   the use of MRI.
  B   stereotactic biopsy.
  C   stereotactic debulking.
  D   the use of dexamethasone.
  E   CSF diversion.

441. An acoustic neuroma
  A   is a neurofibroma rather than a neurilemmoma.
  B   is the underlying cause of Menière's syndrome.
  C   causes tinnitus.
  D   erodes the internal auditory meatus.
  E   causes loss of the corneal reflex.

442. Tumours of the pituitary body include those that are
A   basophil.
B   acidophil.
C   chromophobe.
D   craniopharyngiomas.
E   neurofibromas.

443. Recognised associations with congenital hydrocephalus include
A   myelomeningocele.
B   Budd-Chiari syndrome.
C   failure of development of the arachnoid villi.
D   a cerebral tumour.
E   stenosis of the aqueduct of Sylvius.

444. In the treatment of hydrocephalus
A   a tumour, if the cause of the obstruction, is removed if possible.
B   intracranial shunts may be used for obstruction of the aqueduct of Sylvius.
C   a ventricular shunt into the pleural cavity makes use of the Holter valve.
D   a ventriculoatrial shunt does not require the use of a valve.
E   a ventriculoatrial shunt tube is introduced via the common facial vein.

445. Clinical features characteristic of subarachnoid haemorrhage include
A   sudden severe headache.
B   sudden loss of consciousness.
C   oculomotor nerve palsy.
D   Bell's palsy.
E   Brown-Séquard lesion.

446. With subarachnoid haemorrhage
A   the symptoms can be confused with those due to meningitis.
B   and delay in imaging, antibiotics should be given empirically.
C   calcium antagonists confer benefit.
D   therapeutic embolism is contraindicated.
E   the gamma knife can be effective.

447. Epilepsy

    A   is relatively uncommon in the general population.

    B   is related to the discovery of the use of ECT.

    C   should be investigated by the use of MR imaging.

    D   requires oral anticonvulsant therapy as first line management.

    E   when due to hippocampal sclerosis is not an indication for surgery.

Chapter 9

The eye and orbit
Face, palate, lips
Maxillofacial injuries
The mouth, cheek, tongue
Teeth and gums, jaws, nose, ear
Salivary glands

448. A meibomian cyst
- A   occurs on either the upper or lower lid.
- B   is a granulomatous inflammation of a meibomian gland.
- C   is known as a hordeolum.
- D   characteristically is painful.
- E   is best treated by excision.

449. A retinoblastoma
- A   is a type of ganglioneuroma.
- B   is a malignant undifferentiated tumour.
- C   can be hereditary.
- D   does not metastasise.
- E   can be treated by radiotherapy.

450. A hyphaema is
- A   lymphoedema of the face.
- B   a blue naevus.
- C   haemorrhage into the frontal sinus.
- D   blood in the anterior chamber of the eye.
- E   an angioma.

451. In the differential diagnosis and management of the 'acute red eye'
- A   a drop of fluorescein will show up corneal ulceration.
- B   conjunctivitis does not affect vision.
- C   steroid drops are used for keratitis.
- D   there is an exudate in the anterior chamber and the pupil is notched in glaucoma.
- E   the vomiting in glaucoma can be mistaken as a symptom of an acute abdominal emergency.

452. Keratitis
- A is associated with herpes simplex infection.
- B can follow herpes zoster.
- C causes vitreous detachment.
- D can present as a dendritic ulcer.
- E can be caused by an injection of penicillin.

453. Causes of loss of vision include
- A cranial arteritis.
- B episcleritis.
- C retinal detachment.
- D central retinal vein obstruction.
- E ectropion.

454. Concerning injuries to the eye
- A the pain and photophobia caused by arc welding flash are due to ultraviolet radiation.
- B alkali burns are not serious and respond to simple irrigation.
- C a contusion of the eye may cause a vitreous haemorrhage known as a hyphaema.
- D laceration of the eyelids with bleeding coming from beneath the lids suggests the possibility of a perforating eye injury.
- E an injured eye may have to be enucleated to prevent sympathetic ophthalmia.

455. Sympathetic ophthalmia is
- A conjunctivitis in both eyes due to injury.
- B subconjunctival haemorrhage due to a fractured base of skull.
- C infective (contagious) conjunctivitis.
- D an autoimmune reaction causing blindness in a normal eye following injury of the other eye.
- E part of Horner's syndrome.

456. Acanthosis is
- A an inflammation of the inner canthus of the eye.
- B a proliferation of the prickle cell layer.
- C a cylindroma.
- D leucoplakia of the anus.
- E   aphthous ulceration of the tongue.

457. In infants with cleft lip and cleft palate

A the condition can be familial.
B clefts on the left outnumber those on the right.
C cleft lip interferes with feeding.
D cleft palate interferes with the ability to learn to speak vowels.
E some degree of deafness can occur in those with a cleft palate.

458. In the treatment of cleft lip and cleft palate

A both should be repaired at the age of two years.
B the object with cleft lip is to obtain closure without shortening the upper lip.
C the object with cleft palate is to achieve adequate speech and dentition.
D the repair in cleft palate means suturing both nasal and pharyngeal layers after suitable tension-releasing procedures.
E if the premaxilla is unfused and juts out it has to be excised before repair can be carried out.

459. A preauricular sinus

A is a type of pilonidal sinus.
B can be bilateral.
C is found on the root of the helix or on the tragus.
D is cured by incision and being allowed to heal from the deeper layers.
E can be mistaken for a tuberculous sinus.

460. Treacher Collins' syndrome is associated with

A macrocheilia.
B loss of neural crest cells.
C mandibular prognathism.
D bat ears.
E antimongoloid slant to the palpebral fissure.

461. Lateral swellings of the palate include

A a nasolabial cyst.
B an apical cyst.
C a salivary tumour.
D carcinoma of the maxilla.
E Epstein's pearls.

462. Epiphora is
A   an epiphenomenon of a cerebral tumour.
B   cerebrospinal fluid running from the nose after a fracture of the anterior fossa.
C   an abnormal overflow of tears due to obstruction of the lachrymal duct.
D   eversion of the lower eyelid following injury.
E   a hare lip.

463. Chancre of the lip
A   appears first as bluish-black spots.
B   develops as a painless clean ulcer.
C   imparts a button-like sensation to the examining fingers.
D   produces hard shotty submandibular lymph nodes.
E   is also known as perleche.

464. Carcinoma of the lip
A   if occurring at the angle of the mouth, tends to be more malignant in behaviour than carcinoma of the upper or lower lip.
B   can be confused with a keratoacanthoma.
C   is curable by surgery.
D   is radioresistant.
E   carries a 40% five-year survival rate if seen in its early stages.

465. In a motor accident a young woman has been thrown forward through the windscreen as she has not been wearing a seat belt, therefore
A   the immediate danger is blood loss.
B   the patient is transported supine in the ambulance.
C   there is usually a lot of blood to be seen and this accounts for the shock.
D   excision of dead facial tissue is reduced to a minimum.
E   suture of the skin alone will suffice.

466. One of the types of fracture of the maxilla is suggested by
A   the type of accident.
B   fish face deformity.
C   open bite deformity.
D   diplopia.
E   CSF rhinorrhoea.

94

467. A depressed fractured malar bone and zygomatic arch

   A   can cause diplopia.
   B   is associated with infraorbital anaesthesia.
   C   is associated with a palpable notch of the infraorbital margin.
   D   is treated conservatively.
   E   if compound, is reduced with Walsham's forceps.

468. In cases of fractured nose

   A   swelling often hinders the diagnosis.
   B   delay in treatment, even by a few days, prejudices against a good result.
   C   reduction is usually undertaken under local anaesthesia.
   D   Asch's forceps are used to disimpact the fragments.
   E   Walsham's forceps are used to straighten the septum.

469. In fracture of the mandible

   A   obtaining correct occlusion is of secondary importance in management.
   B   an interdental splint can be used.
   C   teeth on each side of the fracture should be extracted.
   D   the fracture is of the 'closed' type.
   E   delayed union is uncommon.

470. Conditions associated with stomatitis include

   A   vitamin B deficiency.
   B   lupus vulgaris.
   C   lichen planus.
   D   lead poisoning
   E   kwashiorkor.

471. In aphthous stomatitis

   A   telangiectasia occurs.
   B   ulcers can be large and deep.
   C   herpetiform ulcers appear in crops.
   D   Behçet's syndrome can be present.
   E   Reiter's syndrome can be present.

472. The forms in which oral infection with *Candida albicans* appear include

   A   the hyperkeratotic.
   B   the atrophic.
   C   the pseudomembranous.
   D   herpes labialis.
   E   herpangina.

473. **Vincent's acute gingivitis and stomatitis**
   A   is partly due to a spirochaetal infection.
   B   causes angina if affecting the tonsils.
   C   is a recognised complication of cheilosis.
   D   can begin from a partly erupted wisdom tooth.
   E   leads to rhagades.

474. **Ludwig's angina is due to**
   A   a type of coronary artery spasm.
   B   oesophageal spasm.
   C   retropharyngeal infection.
   D   a virulent infection of the cellular tissues around the sub-mandibular salivary gland.
   E   infection with candida.

475. **Cancrum oris**
   A   is due to herpes simplex virus infection.
   B   begins on the gums.
   C   spreads through the whole thickness of the cheek.
   D   unless treated promptly is fatal.
   E   is complicated on healing by the formation of rhagedes.

476. **A ranula is a**
   A   type of epulis.
   B   forked uvula.
   C   sublingual thyroid.
   D   thyroglossal cyst.
   E   cystic swelling in the floor of the mouth.

477. **Lingual dermoids**
   A   produce an opaque swelling.
   B   can be filled with a doughy mass of keratin.
   C   can be filled with mucus.
   D   if median, bulge downwards submentally when the mouth is closed.
   E   if lateral, are derived from the second branchial pouch.

478. **Carcinoma of the cheek**
   A   characteristically is columnar-celled.
   B   can follow a candida-infected speckled leucoplakia.
   C   has a recognised association with chewing gum.
   D   has a recognised association with chewing betel nut.
   E   has a recognised association with geographic tongue.

479. Geographic tongue
A develops as small ulcers near the tip.
B lesions spread and recede in an irregular fashion.
C is a form of lichen planus.
D is premalignant.
E is associated with congenital heart defects.

480. Features characteristic of speckled leucoplakia of the tongue include
A hyperkeratosis.
B plasma cell infiltration within dermal papillae.
C clinically, a paint-like white patch.
D a moist slimy lesion.
E dyskeratosis.

481. Included in the causes of leucoplakia are
A smoking.
B sharp edges of teeth.
C spirit drinking.
D spice chewing.
E candidiasis.

482. The stages of leucoplakia include
A hyperkeratosis.
B elongation of the rete pegs.
C dyskeratosis.
D lichen planus.
E loss of keratinised layer.

483. Ulcers of the tongue
A characteristically follow Ludwig's angina.
B if painful with overhung margins can be due to tuberculosis.
C only occur in the tertiary stage of syphilis.
D can occur in whooping cough.
E are the recognised cause of glossodynia.

484. Carcinoma of the tongue is predisposed to by
A alcohol abuse.
B amyloidosis.
C chewing khat.
D chewing betel nut.
E hairy tongue.

485. **The presentation of carcinoma of the tongue includes**
   A   an oval raised papillated plaque with white keratin flecks on the surface.
   B   a lobulated indurated mass.
   C   a deep fissure.
   D   snail-track ulceration.
   E   Hutchinson's wart.

486. **The management of carcinoma of the tongue includes**
   A   an adequate biopsy.
   B   excision biopsy.
   C   oral hygiene.
   D   serological tests for syphilis.
   E   radiotherapy.

487. **In a patient with carcinoma of the tongue**
   A   ankyloglossia occurs when the cancer begins on the dorsum of the tongue.
   B   it may simply present with a lump in the neck.
   C   alteration of the voice is an early feature of carcinoma situated at the back of the tongue.
   D   a lesion which begins on one side of the anterior two-thirds of the tongue soon spreads across the midline to the other side.
   E   the lymphatics draining the anterior two-thirds of the tongue and the floor of the mouth transverse the periosteum of the mandible in many instances.

488. **When clinically malignant lymph nodes appear in the neck**
   A   the site of the primary is easy to find.
   B   the testis could be the primary site.
   C   palpable cervical lymph nodes draining a primary tumour are not necessarily involved by growth.
   D   adherence of a node or tumour to the mandible is a contra-indication to surgery.
   E   when the cervical lymph nodes are fixed it is helpful to make an incision directly over them to obtain a biopsy.

489. **In classical block dissection of the neck**
  A   the sternomastoid is detached from its lower attachment and resutured at the end of the operation.
  B   a length of the internal jugular vein is removed.
  C   the common cartoid artery is tied.
  D   the contents of the submental triangle are removed.
  E   the cervical branch of the facial nerve is preserved.

490. **The commando operation is**
  A   abdominoperineal excision of the rectum for carcinoma.
  B   disarticulation of the hip for gas gangrene in the leg.
  C   extended radical mastectomy.
  D   excision of carcinoma of the tongue, the floor of the mouth, part of the jaw and lymph nodes *en bloc*.
  E   the delayed primary suture of missile wounds.

491. **The ameloblastoma**
  A   can be cystic.
  B   commonly occurs in the maxilla.
  C   characteristically is a painful lesion.
  D   can be excised.
  E   metastasises to the lungs.

492. **The impacted lower third molar (wisdom) tooth is associated with**
  A   caries in the second molar.
  B   pericoronitis.
  C   giant cell granuloma.
  D   food packing.
  E   lateral dentigerous cyst.

493. **Recognised consequences of alveolar abscess include**
  A   parapharyngeal abscess.
  B   Vincent's angina.
  C   submental sinus.
  D   cavernous sinus thrombosis.
  E   facial sinus.

494. If a patient aged 50 has osteomyelitis of the jaw

A   an injudicious tooth extraction may have been performed under local anaesthetic.

B   the mandible is less affected than the maxilla because it has a better blood supply.

C   an early x-ray will confirm the diagnosis.

D   operation is necessary to relieve tension.

E   bone recovery is poor.

495. Dental caries increases the risk of morbidity from surgical procedures. It favours the occurrence of

A   stomatitis.

B   parotitis.

C   bacteraemia.

D   lung abscess.

E   acute pyelonephritis.

496. Lumps on the gum include

A   Paget's disease of the jaw.

B   giant cell granuloma.

C   fibrous epulis.

D   pregnancy epulis.

E   pyogenic granuloma.

497. Cystic lesions of the jaw include

A   dental cyst.

B   nasopalatine cyst.

C   dentigerous cyst.

D   Paget's disease.

E   cementifying fibromas.

498. A giant cell tumour of the jaw

A   is malignant.

B   histologically resembles giant epulis.

C   can enlarge alarmingly during pregnancy.

D   is associated with aneursymal bone cyst.

E   can respond satisfactorily to calcitonin therapy.

499. Of the malignant tumours affecting the mandible
- A a squamous cell carcinoma is the commonest.
- B the torus palatinus is a variety.
- C Paget's disease can be a precursor.
- D one type can be histiocytosis X.
- E adenocarcinoma can be present.

500. The clinical features of carcinoma of the maxillary antrum include
- A toothache.
- B free bleeding on proof puncture of the antrum.
- C epiphora.
- D entropion.
- E proptosis.

501. The Caldwell-Luc operation is appropriate for
- A removing nasal polypi.
- B cataract.
- C draining intractable purulent maxillary sinusitis.
- D closing an oral-antral fistula.
- E glaucoma.

502. Epistaxis
- A is commonly epistaxis digitorum.
- B usually comes from veins in Little's area.
- C is a feature of hypertension.
- D if coming from the front of the nose the immediate treatment is to pack the nostrils.
- E sometimes requires arterial ligation.

503. A deflected nasal septum is treated by
- A inserting a prosthesis.
- B removal.
- C straightening.
- D submucous resection.
- E antrostomy.

504. Otitis externa
- A is also known as telephonist's ear.
- B is usually caused by trauma to and infection of a sebaceous cyst.
- C can be caused by seborrhoea.
- D is treated by being syringed daily.
- E requires that the feet be inspected and treated if relevant.

505. **Carcinoma of the pinna**
   A   is an extension of carcinoma of the auditory canal.
   B   is known as Singapore ear.
   C   is a basal-celled carcinoma.
   D   is best treated by radiotherapy.
   E   may require the ear to be cut off.

506. **Glue ear**
   A   is synonymous with seromucinous otitis media.
   B   affects those with large infected adenoids.
   C   is also synonymous with acute otitis media.
   D   is common in children with a cleft palate.
   E   is characteristically painless.

507. **Acute otitis media**
   A   can present with vomiting.
   B   inevitably causes acute mastoiditis.
   C   causes perforation of the eardrum.
   D   is synonymous with 'telephonist's ear'.
   E   inevitably requires myringotomy.

508. **In acute otitis media**
   A   it is secondary to furunculosis of the ear.
   B   it presents with painful deaf ear.
   C   antibiotics are helpful only if given early and as a full course.
   D   myringotomy is performed if pus appears.
   E   chronic otitis media is the usual complication.

509. **Unsafe CSOM**
   A   is characteristically associated with cholesteatoma.
   B   exhibits a retraction pocket in the attic.
   C   is usually dry.
   D   is treated by myringotomy.
   E   can be followed by facial palsy.

510. **Serous otitis media**
   A   is synonymous with glue ear.
   B   commonly occurs in children.
   C   causes conduction deafness.
   D   is related to flying.
   E   causes Menière's syndrome.

511. The recognised immediate management of a ruptured ear drum includes
   A   eardrops.
   B   daily examination.
   C   insertion of a grommet tube.
   D   myringotomy.
   E   syringing with saline.

512. Menière's disease can be treated by
   A   a plastic operation.
   B   a prosthesis.
   C   stapedectomy.
   D   insertion of a grommet.
   E   labyrinthectomy.

513. Pes anserinus is
   A   syndactyly affecting the toes.
   B   club foot.
   C   the arrangement of the cervical plexus in the neck.
   D   a description of the arrangement of the facial nerve.
   E   a flat foot.

514. Regarding the anatomy of the salivary glands
   A   the parotid gland lies wholly deep to the facial nerve.
   B   the socia parotidis lies below and behind the ear over the mastoid process.
   C   the parotid duct opens in the mouth opposite the upper canine tooth.
   D   the submandibular gland lies in the submental triangle.
   E   the submandibular gland empties by several small ducts into the floor of the mouth.

515. In the anatomy of the submandibular salivary gland
   A   the facial artery lies intimately within the gland.
   B   the lingual nerve is enclosed within the fascial sheath of the gland.
   C   the deep part of the gland lies on the hyoglossus in relation to the hypoglossal nerve.
   D   the submandibular ganglion is attached below the gland.
   E   the submandibular duct emerges from the lower pole of the gland.

516. Acute parotitis

A may be due to non-specific bacterial infection.
B may be due to the Coxsackie A virus.
C is likely in the postoperative period following major surgery.
D requires immediate incision.
E with pus formation is immediately fluctuant.

517. Concerning salivary calculi

A submandibular stones in the duct are removed via the floor of the mouth.
B submandibular stones in the gland are extracted from the gland through an incision in the neck.
C parotid calculi are more common than submandibular calculi.
D salivary stones contain calcium carbonate.
E a parotid duct stone causes cysts of the parotid.

518. The treatment of submandibular calculus lying within the duct is to

A dilate the duct.
B remove the stone by making an opening in the duct.
C slit open the duct at the papilla.
D remove the gland.
E ligature the duct.

519. In relation to salivary strictures and fistulas

A any submandibular duct stricture is an indication for removal of the gland.
B multiple parotid strictures are pathognomonic of Sjögren's syndrome.
C a fistula from a divided parotid gland will usually heal by granulation.
D a fistula from a divided parotid duct must be explored.
E parotidectomy is necessary if the parotid duct fistula cannot be repaired successfully.

520. In the management of a pleomorphic adenoma of the parotid

A a biopsy is taken.
B operation is advised.
C the tumour is enucleated.
D partial parotidectomy with conservation of the facial nerve is preferred.
E postoperative radiotherapy is given.

521. A Warthin's tumour is
A an adenolymphoma of the parotid gland.
B a pleomorphic adenoma of the parotid.
C a cylindroma.
D a carcinoma of the parotid.
E a carcinoma of the submandibular salivary gland.

522. Regarding the treatment of a clinically malignant parotid tumour
A the lesion is usually radiosensitive.
B if operation is advised the facial nerve should be preserved.
C a frozen section during operation is helpful before any irrevocable mutilating step is taken.
D excision of the mandible is mandatory.
E the prognosis is good.

523. Recognised features of Sjögren's syndrome include
A dry eyes.
B rheumatoid arthritis.
C psoriasis.
D proptosis.
E a dry mouth.

524. Frey's syndrome
A is only manifest on chewing food.
B includes facial sweating of skin innervated by the facial nerve.
C can follow parotidectomy.
D can follow birth trauma.
E can be alleviated by use of a 'roll on' antiperspirant.

Chapter 10

The pharynx
The larynx
The neck

525. **The anatomy of the tonsil includes the fact that**
    A   the intratonsillar cleft is erroneously called the supratonsillar fossa.
    B   it is related medially to the inferior constrictor muscle.
    C   it is pierced superiorly by the tonsillar artery.
    D   the paratonsillar vein is in close lateral relationship.
    E   innervation via the glossopharyngeal nerve accounts for pain in the ear in tonsillitis.

526. **The usual cause of acute follicular tonsillitis is infection with**
    A   *Streptococcus pyogenes.*
    B   *Staphylococcus aureus.*
    C   *Klebsiella.*
    D   *Candida.*
    E   *Aspergillus.*

527. **If a patient has a quinsy**
    A   he or she is usually between eight and 18 years old.
    B   it is a retropharyngeal abscess.
    C   saliva dribbles from the mouth.
    D   the uvula is displaced.
    E   a general anaesthetic is essential for operation.

528. **Clinical manifestations relating to a pharyngeal pouch include**
    A   in stage 1, no symptoms.
    B   in stage 2, regurgitation.
    C   in stage 2, lung abscess.
    D   in stage 3, cardiospasm.
    E   in stage 3, dysphagia lusoria.

529. **Angiofibroma of the nasopharynx**
    A   is a benign tumour.
    B   never metastasises.
    C   is highly destructive.
    D   causes a 'frog face'.
    E   occurs in boys.

530. **Malignant tumours of the nasopharynx**
   A   mostly arise in the 'supratonsillar' fossa of Rosenmüller.
   B   in the UK occur especially where furniture is made.
   C   do not involve cranial nerves.
   D   by the time a diagnosis is made, 70% of the patients have enlarged cervical nodes.
   E   are spindle-celled sarcomas.

531. **Recognised clinical features of carcinoma of the nasopharynx include**
   A   trigeminal neuralgia.
   B   conductive deafness without pain in the ear.
   C   secretory otitis media.
   D   immobility of the soft palate.
   E   Plummer-Vinson syndrome.

532. **In the presence of a malignant tumour of the nasopharynx, Trotter's triad includes**
   A   persistent nasal catarrh.
   B   epistaxis.
   C   pain in the side of the head.
   D   elevation of the homolateral soft palate.
   E   conductive deafness.

533. **A malignant tumour in the sinus piriformis**
   A   can present as an enlarged lymph node behind the angle of the jaw.
   B   causes pain in the hip.
   C   causes pain in the hand.
   D   presents with pain in the mandible.
   E   causes swelling of the maxillary antrum.

534. **Cryosurgery is recognised as useful in the treatment of**
   A   angiofibromas.
   B   haemangiomas.
   C   painful uncontrolled cancers.
   D   piles.
   E   perniosis.

535. **Regarding acute oedema of the glottis**
   A   it is oedema of the vocal cords.
   B   some cases are due to angioneurotic oedema.
   C   dysphagia may be present.
   D   if observed through the laryngoscope it looks like the cervix.
   E   morphine is used to allay stridor.

536. A cricoid hook is used particularly
  A   in thyroidectomy.
  B   in block dissection of the neck.
  C   for retracting the cricothyroid muscle.
  D   in tracheostomy.
  E   for retracting the recurrent laryngeal nerve.

537. Tracheal stenosis
  A   is caused by intratracheal tumours.
  B   commonly follows tracheostomy at the site of the inflatable cuff.
  C   can be treated by incision of the trachea.
  D   is a complication of tuberculosis.
  E   is due to retrosternal goitre.

538. With laryngeal paralysis
  A   the cricothyroid muscle is paralysed after recurrent laryngeal nerve injury.
  B   the vocal fold will be lying in the 'death' position if there is bilateral recurrent laryngeal nerve injury.
  C   a complete unilateral recurrent nerve palsy is an indication for early (one month) endoscopic injection of Teflon paste close to the thyroid cartilage.
  D   tracheostomy is necessary in all cases of bilateral paralysis.
  E   a tracheostomy speaking valve would not be of any value.

539. Malignant tumours of the larynx
  A   are characteristically columnar-celled.
  B   are associated with smoking.
  C   if glottic carry the worst prognosis.
  D   if supraglottic metastasise early.
  E   are not radiosensitive.

540. The right recurrent laryngeal nerve can be damaged by
  A   malignant infiltration of the thyroid gland.
  B   operation on the thyroid gland.
  C   operation on a persistent ductus arteriosus.
  D   secondary lymph nodes from carcinoma of the bronchus.
  E   pressure of an aneurysm of the aortic arch.

541. When classical block dissection of the neck is carried out with laryngectomy

A   a length of the internal jugular vein is removed.

B   partial thyroidectomy may have to be included.

C   the sternomastoid is detached from its lower attachment and resutured at the end of the operation.

D   the common carotid artery is ligated.

E   the contents of the supraclavicular triangle should be removed.

542. The anterior triangle of the neck

A   is bounded anteriorly by the median line.

B   is bounded posteriorly by the posterior margin of the sternomastoid.

C   has as its base the upper border of the clavicle.

D   contains the carotid triangle.

E   contains the supraclavicular triangle.

543. A branchial cyst

A   commonly appears between the 20th and 25th years.

B   arises from the vestigial remnants of the fourth branchial cleft.

C   is usually lined by squamous epithelium.

D   does not become inflamed like neighbouring lymph nodes.

E   can be contiguous with a track which passes through the fork of the carotid artery as far as the pharyngeal wall.

544. A cystic hygroma is

A   a type of cavernous haemangioma.

B   a complication of hyperhidrosis.

C   a cystic rodent.

D   brilliantly translucent.

E   a variety of hydradenitis.

545. The 'potato' tumour of the neck is a tumour of

A   sternomastoid muscle.

B   carotid body.

C   thyroid gland.

D   parotid gland.

E   parathyroid gland.

546. **In the supraclavicular triangle the**
A floor includes the scalenus medius muscle.
B subclavian vein is normally prominent.
C first part of the subclavian artery lies in front of the scalenus anterior.
D nerves of the brachial plexus lie above and behind the subclavian artery.
E external jugular vein terminates in the subclavian vein.

547. **Regarding a cervical rib**
A it can always be felt in the neck.
B the bone of the rib is always the cause of the symptoms.
C it can cause ischaemic muscle pain in the forearm.
D trophic changes can occur in the fingers.
E treatment is subperiosteal excision of the rib.

548. **Ludwig's angina**
A is associated with coronary artery spasm.
B is a form of oesophageal spasm.
C is characterised by putrid halitosis.
D is an infection of a closed fascial space.
E untreated is likely to be fatal.

549. **In tuberculous lymphadenitis of the neck**
A the patient may be an elderly woman.
B the bovine bacillus is mostly responsible.
C a primary focus in the lungs may be present.
D the nodes tend to be matted together.
E a collar stud abscess may form.

550. **Characteristic of a carotid body tumour is that**
A the tumour is pulsatile.
B it is easy to dissect from the carotid artery.
C at operation it may well be necessary to use a temporary bypass while a vein graft is being inserted.
D if the internal carotid artery is simply ligated in the removal of the tumour, death or hemiplegia follows in 33% of cases.
E recurrence is unusual after complete resection.

551. **A cold abscess beneath the skin**
   A feels colder than the surrounding skin.
   B is caused by frostbite.
   C should be incised immediately.
   D is treated with penicillin.
   E is due to tuberculosis.

552. **In the carotid triangle**
   A lies the common carotid artery.
   B the external carotid artery lies posterior to the internal carotid.
   C the inferior thyroid artery is a branch of the common carotid artery.
   D the hypoglossal nerve crosses the internal and external carotid arteries.
   E the internal jugular vein is prominent.

553. **The special danger of a carotid body tumour is that it**
   A recurs after excision.
   B is blended with the carotid artery.
   C is blended with the external jugular vein.
   D is radioresistant.
   E has an expansile pulsation.

554. **In the management of secondary carcinoma of the neck**
   A the source and histology of the primary growth must be known.
   B cervical nodes must be excised *en bloc* with a neck primary.
   C if radiotherapy has been used, a subsequent block dissection should not be done.
   D if developing subsequent to successful treatment of a primary, a block dissection can be curative.
   E a bilateral block dissection is best done at the same sitting.

Chapter 11

The thyroid and thyroglossal tract
The parathyroid and adrenal glands

555. **The blood vessels to and from the thyroid including name and branch or tributary include**
    A   the superior thyroid artery, being a branch of the internal carotid artery.
    B   the middle thyroid vein – a tributary of the external jugular vein.
    C   the middle thyroid artery – a branch of the external carotid artery.
    D   the inferior thyroid artery – a branch of the thyrocervical trunk.
    E   the inferior thyroid veins – tributaries of the innominate veins.

556. **A lingual thyroid**
    A   forms a swelling in the upper part of the neck.
    B   is associated with struma ovarii – part of an ectopic ovarian teratoma.
    C   can be excised without any difficulty or hormonal problem.
    D   is likely to shrink if the patient is given L-thyroxine.
    E   is related to the foramen caecum.

557. **The term lateral aberrant thyroid really implies**
    A   congenital aberrant thyroid tissue lateral to the thyroid.
    B   a metastasis in a cervical lymph node from an occult thyroid carcinoma.
    C   a metastasis from carcinoma of the larynx.
    D   a type of branchial cyst.
    E   that a loose piece of thyroid has become implanted in a thyroidectomy scar.

558. **A thyroglossal fistula**
    A   has the internal opening beside the fraenum linguae.
    B   follows inadequate removal of a thyroglossal cyst.
    C   externally has a hood of skin with its concavity upwards.
    D   is lined throughout by squamous epithelium.
    E   occurs in carcinoma of the tongue.

559. **In the operation for thyroglossal fistula**
  A   the track is dissected as it passes behind the hyoid cartilage onwards up the tongue.
  B   the track is dissected as it passes behind, below and in front of the hyoid cartilage.
  C   the middle portion of the hyoid cartilage is excised.
  D   the track is dissected upwards until it enters the mouth close to the frenum of the tongue.
  E   the track is dissected and excised with a central core of lingual muscle extending centrally towards the foramen caecum.

560. **Routine tests for thyroid function include**
  A   total serum T4.
  B   serum alkaline phosphatase.
  C   free serum T3.
  D   serum calcitonin.
  E   TSH.

561. **Myxoedema**
  A   is an advanced form of juvenile hypothyroidism.
  B   is related to thyroidectomy and ^{131}I therapy.
  C   is a cause of carpal tunnel syndrome.
  D   returns a serum T4 below 3.0 µg/100 ml (60 mmol/l)
  E   is treated by potassium iodide.

562. **Regarding simple goitre**
  A   if sporadic it means that it is prevalent in a people or a district.
  B   a diffuse hyperplastic goitre feels firm to hard on palpation.
  C   a nodular goitre tends to be painful.
  D   a nodular goitre may be complicated by a follicular carcinoma.
  E   all types of simple goitre are more common in the female than in the male.

563. **Clinically discrete thyroid swellings**
  A   are termed isolated if in an otherwise impalpable gland.
  B   are termed dominant if in a gland of generalised nodularity.
  C   are rarely malignant if isolated.
  D   if 'hot' on isotope scanning are invariably malignant.
  E   should be investigated by FNAC.

564. **Clinical criteria used in assessing the desirability of operation for discrete thyroid swellings include**
   A   purely hardness of texture.
   B   evidence of recurrent nerve paralysis.
   C   enlarged internal jugular lymph nodes.
   D   a swelling in a teenager of either sex.
   E   a swelling in a male patient.

565. **Retrosternal goitre**
   A   usually arises from ectopic thyroid tissue.
   B   can be of the plunging type.
   C   can cause a 'scabbard' trachea.
   D   is treated in the first instance by radio-iodine.
   E   may have to be removed piecemeal.

566. **In a patient with a retrosternal goitre**
   A   a ^{131}I scan may help to distinguish a retrosternal from a mediastinal tumour.
   B   dysphagia is common.
   C   recurrent nerve paralysis is common.
   D   myasthenia gravis occurs.
   E   the blood supply to the goitre comes from the neck.

567. **Concerning the clinicopathological features of hyperthyroidism**
   A   it may occur at any age.
   B   enophthalmos is a characteristic feature.
   C   cardiac arrhythmias are superimposed on the sinus tachycardia.
   D   myasthenia gravis is a late feature.
   E   histology reveals acini lined by flattened cuboidal epithelium filled with homogeneous colloid.

568. **True exophthalmos**
   A   is associated with proptosis of the eye.
   B   is due to retrobulbar infiltration with fluid and round cells.
   C   associated upper eyelid spasm and retraction may be improved by β-adrenergic drugs as eye drops.
   D   can be complicated by chemosis.
   E   can proceed to a malignant variety which causes secondary deposits in the liver ('beware the glass eye and the large liver').

569. **Pretibial myxoedema**
   A   is a thickening of the skin by a mucin-like deposit.
   B   may be cyanotic when cold.
   C   is an occasional feature of myxoedema.
   D   is associated with low levels of LATS.
   E   can be associated with clubbing of the fingers and toes.

570. **Drugs used in the treatment of thyrotoxicosis include**
   A   propylthiouracil.
   B   propranolol.
   C   iodides in the long term.
   D   beclomethasone diproprionate.
   E   carbimazole.

571. **The disadvantage of using radio-iodine to treat thyrotoxicosis is that**
   A   drug therapy is prolonged.
   B   an indefinite follow-up is essential.
   C   there is a progressive incidence of thyroid insufficiency.
   D   it has to be avoided under the age of 45.
   E   subsequent malignancy is not excluded.

572. **Action in the preparation of a patient for thyroidectomy for thyro-toxicosis includes**
   A   the patient being brought into a euthyroid state.
   B   recording changes in weight and sleeping pulse rate.
   C   the use of chlorpropamide for preparation.
   D   the use of potassium perchlorate with Lugol's iodine (or potassium iodide).
   E   using propranolol which does not act on the thyroid itself and has to be carried on postoperatively.

573. **The steps in the operation of subtotal thyroidectomy include**
   A   general anaesthesia by an endotracheal tube.
   B   an H-shaped incision.
   C   dividing the middle thyroid artery.
   D   identification of the course of the recurrent laryngeal nerves.
   E   haemostasis by diathermy of veins leaving the thyroid.

574. **The immediate postoperative complications of thyroidectomy include**
   A   secondary haemorrhage.
   B   laryngeal oedema.
   C   hypothyroidism.
   D   keloid scarring.
   E   surgical emphysema.

575. **The right recurrent laryngeal nerve can be damaged by**
   A malignant infiltration of the thyroid gland.
   B operation on the thyroid gland.
   C operation on a persistent ductus arteriosus.
   D secondary lymph nodes from carcinoma of the bronchus.
   E pressure by an aneurysm of the aortic arch.

576. **Primary malignant tumours of the thyroid include those that are**
   A squamous.
   B papillary.
   C columnar.
   D follicular.
   E basaloid.

577. **The presentation of carcinoma of the thyroid includes**
   A earache.
   B hoarseness of the voice.
   C a pulsating bone tumour.
   D the sex ratio being three males to one female.
   E hyperthyroidism.

578. **Recognised associations of medullary carcinoma of the thyroid include**
   A other members of the family being affected.
   B constipation being a feature in 30% of cases.
   C a phaeochromocytoma.
   D neuromas on the tongue.
   E hormone dependency.

579. **Total thyroidectomy**
   A is indicated for papillary carcinoma.
   B is indicated for medullary carcinoma.
   C is often impossible for anaplastic carcinoma.
   D includes the removal of all the parathyroid glands in close relationship with the thyroid.
   E necessarily means the division of both recurrent laryngeal nerves.

580. **Thyroiditis is**
   A caused by a virus, if granulomatous.
   B associated with pernicious anaemia.
   C associated with malignant lymphoma.
   D is commonest in men after prostatectomy.
   E is a type of struma ovarii.

116

581. Features consistent with a diagnosis of Hashimoto's disease include
A   a painful gland.
B   hyperthyroidism.
C   hypothyroidism.
D   swelling localised to one lobe.
E   a high 48-hour PB^{131}I uptake test result in the absence of a previous thyroidectomy or radio-iodine therapy.

582. Hashimoto's disease is
A   chronic lymphocytic thyroiditis.
B   an autoimmune thyroiditis.
C   an infiltrating fibrosis of the thyroid and the adjacent muscles.
D   associated with mumps.
E   a parathyroid tumour.

583. Regarding the parathyroid glands
A   they are found in the thyroid rarely.
B   the 'chief' cells produce parathormone.
C   parathormone stimulates osteoblastic activity.
D   parathormone reduces the renal tubular reabsorption of phosphate.
E   calcitonin is secreted by the oxyphil cells of the parathyroid.

584. Regarding parathyroid tetany
A   it is a common complication of subtotal thyroidectomy.
B   the symptoms appear immediately on recovery from the anaesthetic.
C   acrocyanosis occurs.
D   symptoms can be relieved by 10–20 ml of 10% solution of calcium gluconate.
E   the level of serum calcium should be estimated daily as a guide to calcium dosage.

585. The clinical features related to hyperparathyroidism include
A   risus sardonicus.
B   tetany.
C   personality changes.
D   lumpy and bumpy lips.
E   hypothermia.

586. **After operation for hyperparathyroidism**
  A   renal stones disappear.
  B   bones recalcify.
  C   psychiatric patients improve.
  D   hyperparathyroidism recurs in a small minority of patients.
  E   hypothyroidism is a characteristic complication.

587. **Hyperparathyroidism is associated with**
  A   corneal calcification.
  B   stones.
  C   abdominal groans.
  D   hypertension.
  E   vitreous detachment.

588. **The causes of hypercalcaemia include**
  A   parathyroid adenoma.
  B   acute pancreatitis.
  C   multiple myeloma.
  D   phaeochromocytoma.
  E   sarcoidosis.

589. **Concerning the adrenal glands**
  A   they attain nearly adult proportions at birth.
  B   the right adrenal is semilunar in shape.
  C   on the left side, the adrenal vein enters into the left renal vein.
  D   the left gland is a little larger than the right.
  E   they are exocrine glands.

590. **The adrenal cortex**
  A   contains the glomerular zone.
  B   contains the acanthotic layer.
  C   contains the reticular zone.
  D   makes androgens.
  E   is inhibited by ACTH.

591. **Tests relating to adrenocortical activity include those named as**
  A   VMA.
  B   MIBG.
  C   TRC.
  D   ACTH.
  E   SYNACTHEN.

592. Aldosterone
  A   is a mineralocorticoid.
  B   regulates water balance.
  C   stimulates sodium excretion.
  D   stimulates potassium retention.
  E   facilitates gluconeogenesis.

593. Hydrocortisone
  A   is a glucocorticoid.
  B   diminishes allergic reaction.
  C   influences the distribution of body fat.
  D   increases the catabolism of proteins.
  E   stimulates the development of fibroblasts.

594. Acute hypocorticism is recognised to be associated with
  A   haemorrhage.
  B   oestrogen withdrawal.
  C   syphilis.
  D   meningitis.
  E   tuberculosis.

595. The clinical features of Addison's disease include
  A   hyperglycaemia.
  B   hypertension.
  C   loss of body hair.
  D   muscular weakness.
  E   pigmentation of the mouth.

596. Types of hypercorticism include
  A   Conn's syndrome.
  B   Simmond's disease.
  C   Addison's disease.
  D   Cushing's syndrome.
  E   adrenogenital syndrome.

597. The clinical features of Cushing's disease include
  A   kyphoscoliosis.
  B   limb muscle atrophy.
  C   acne.
  D   glycosuria.
  E   Hippocratic facies.

598. Conn's syndrome is associated with
A a secretory adenoma of the parathyroids.
B polyuria.
C right ventricular hypertrophy.
D tetany.
E low serum potassium level.

599. In Cushing's syndrome
A there is chronic hypocorticism.
B there is an excessive production of glucocorticoids.
C there is a malignant adrenal neoplasm present in about 50% of cases.
D one-third of the patients have a basophil tumour of the adrenal.
E there is water retention.

600. Phaeochromocytoma
A is bilateral in about 15% of cases.
B produces noradrenaline.
C is recognised to be present in all patients under 60 years who present with sustained arterial hypertension.
D is treated definitively with antihypertensive drugs.
E causes pigmentation of the skin.

601. Phaeochromocytoma
A can occur at the aortic bifurcation.
B if extrarenal is more likely to be benign.
C is pink-tan in colour.
D contains chromaffin granules.
E is associated with MEN IIa and MEN IIb.

602. A patient undergoing an operation for removal of a phaeochromo-cytoma
A is hypovolaemic.
B will suffer a surge of circulating catecholamine.
C will have sustained hypertension after removal of the tumour.
D can be protected by the use of phenoxybenzamine with a β-blocker.
E should have the main adrenal vein ligated before removal of the tumour.

603. In a child with neuroblastoma of the adrenal

A   the disease begins in the cortex.

B   the age of the child is most likely to be over seven years.

C   a left-sided primary tends to give rise to secondaries in the orbit and skull.

D   a right-sided primary tends to give rise to large liver metastases.

E   spontaneous remission is known to occur.

Chapter 12

The breast

604. Concerning the lymphatic system draining the breast
- **A** there is a free communication between the subclavicular and supraclavicular lymph nodes.
- **B** the lymph nodes along the internal mammary chain are involved in about half the cases in which the axillary nodes are implicated by carcinoma.
- **C** there is no subareolar plexus.
- **D** some lymph nodes lie between the greater and lesser pectoral muscles.
- **E** cancer cells can spread retrogradely.

605. Of the investigations employed in the diagnosis of breast lesions
- **A** mammography submits the breast to high amperage x-rays.
- **B** ductography is a painless and useful imaging technique.
- **C** ultrasonography can distinguish cystic from solid tumours.
- **D** cytology derived from multiple passes of a 23 gauge needle with syringe suction is a painless procedure without anaesthesia.
- **E** FNAC is totally reliable.

606. Retraction of the nipple
- **A** is always unilateral.
- **B** is characteristic of Paget's disease.
- **C** is associated with duct ectasia.
- **D** if recent can be due to a chancre.
- **E** can be caused by fat necrosis.

607. A cracked nipple is
- **A** due to a syphilitic chancre.
- **B** a cause of a retention cyst of a gland of Montgomery.
- **C** Paget's disease of the nipple.
- **D** a forerunner of a breast abscess.
- **E** likely in the puerperium.

608. A blood-stained discharge from the nipple indicates
- **A** the likely presence of breast abscess.
- **B** fibroadenoma.
- **C** duct papilloma.
- **D** duct ectasia.
- **E** fat necrosis of the breast.

609. **Fat necrosis of the breast**
   A   occurs when the patient also has acute pancreatitis.
   B   causes retraction of the nipple.
   C   is synonymous with Mondor's disease.
   D   is confined to pregnancy.
   E   causes skin dimpling.

610. **The treatment of a breast abscess should include**
   A   incision.
   B   mastectomy.
   C   biopsy.
   D   antibiotics.
   E   inhibition of lactation.

611. **A breast abscess**
   A   can follow mumps.
   B   first goes through a stage of milk engorgement.
   C   goes through a stage of bacterial mastitis.
   D   characteristically is caused by the haemolytic streptococcus.
   E   is necessarily treated by aspiration.

612. **A milk fistula**
   A   occurs in lactating women.
   B   emanates from accessory nipples.
   C   is related to recurrent abscesses of the areolar region.
   D   can be related to duct ectasia.
   E   must be treated in the same way as a low fistula *in ano*.

613. **Tuberculosis of the breast**
   A   can present as an abscess.
   B   spreads to the breast by retrograde lymphatic spread.
   C   tends to occur in nullipara.
   D   causes sinuses with bluish edges.
   E   is treated by mastectomy.

614. **Mondor's disease is**
   A   an obscure type of thrombophlebitis particularly affecting veins of the breast.
   B   lymphoedema of the arm.
   C   chondritis of a costal cartilage.
   D   pectus excavatum.
   E   eczema of the nipple.

615. Mammary duct ectasia is characteristically associated with
  A   blue domed cysts.
  B   plasma cell mastitis.
  C   retraction of the nipple.
  D   bacterial infection.
  E   Paget's disease of the nipple.

616. Duct ectasia of the breast
  A   occurs in young multipara.
  B   means that the ducts are dilated with mucus.
  C   presents with a worm-like swelling extending radially from the nipple.
  D   is associated with periductal inflammation with lymphocytes and plasma cells.
  E   is a premalignant condition.

617. Of the discharges from the nipple, that which is
  A   purulent is diagnostic of duct ectasia.
  B   blood-stained is consistent with duct ectasia.
  C   milk is consistent with hyperthyroidism.
  D   serous is most likely due to fibrocystic disease.
  E   grumous indicates a carcinoma.

618. In a patient with fibroadenosis of the breast
  A   duct papillomatosis may be present.
  B   pregnancy usually produces relief.
  C   the breasts feel nodular and the periphery has a saucer-like edge.
  D   radiotherapy is a useful palliative treatment.
  E   the breasts should be replaced by prosthetic implants.

619. Changes in the breast implied by the term 'mammary dysplasia' include
  A   cyst formation.
  B   metaplasia.
  C   leucoplakia.
  D   epitheliosis.
  E   adenosis.

620. **Non-malignant conditions of the breast include**
 A cystosarcoma phylloides.
 B duct ectasia.
 C giant fibroadenoma.
 D Paget's disease of the nipple.
 E fat necrosis.

621. **Duct papilloma of the breast**
 A commonly occurs in women aged between 35 and 50 years.
 B presents as a cystic swelling felt beneath the areola.
 C is characteristically a single lesion.
 D should be treated by simple mastectomy.
 E becomes a papillary adenocarcinoma.

622. **Massive swellings of the breast include**
 A cystosarcoma phylloides.
 B atrophic scirrhous carcinoma.
 C diffuse hypertrophy.
 D Mondor's disease.
 E Paget's disease of the nipple.

623. **The difference between eczema and Paget's disease of the nipple is that eczema**
 A is unilateral.
 B is related to lactation.
 C manifests vesicles.
 D does not respond to simple treatment.
 E is associated with a minute duct carcinoma within the breast.

624. **Clinical signs supporting an early diagnosis of carcinoma of the breast include**
 A a prickling sensation in a breast lump.
 B *peau d'orange*.
 C brawny arm.
 D cancer *en cuirasse*.
 E palpable axillary nodes.

625. **In carcinoma of the breast**
 A the malignant cells transgress the internal elastic lamina of a duct.
 B the medullary (anaplastic) type feels stony hard.
 C the atrophic scirrhous type occurs in younger women.
 D pain is characteristically an early feature.
 E it is virtually impossible clinically to distinguish a duct papilloma from a duct carcinoma.

626. **In the generally accepted clinical staging of carcinoma of the breast (Manchester staging)**
   A in Stage I an area of adherence to the skin smaller than the periphery of the tumour does not affect staging.
   B in Stage II axillary nodes are palpable and immobile.
   C the absence of palpable nodes means that carcinoma has not spread to them.
   D if the tumour is fixed to the pectoral muscle but not to the chest wall it is nevertheless Stage IV.
   E cancer *en cuirasse* is included in Stage IV.

627. **In the clinical staging of carcinoma of the breast by the TNM classification, a stating of $T_2N_2M_1$ includes the fact that**
   A the tumour is more than 5 cm in diameter.
   B skin is tethered to the tumour.
   C axillary nodes are palpable but movable.
   D there is oedema of the arm.
   E there are no metastases.

628. **A macroscopic characteristic of a cancer of the breast is that**
   A the growth cuts like an unripe pear.
   B both surfaces are usually concave.
   C the colour of the cut surface is grey.
   D the remains of a capsule will be found.
   E cysts are prevalent.

629. **In the operation of radical mastectomy (Halsted's operation)**
   A an area of skin 4–6 inches in diameter is removed.
   B the nipple can be retained or transplanted to a new site.
   C the latissimus dorsi is removed.
   D the pectoralis minor muscle is retained.
   E the long thoracic nerve should be spared.

630. **In a 'Patey' type of mastectomy the *en bloc* removal of the tissues include the**
   A whole breast.
   B the nipple.
   C the pectoralis major.
   D the clavipectoral fascia.
   E the third and fourth anterior intercostal lymph nodes.

631. Of the adjuvant therapy to operation for carcinoma of the breast

 A the tamoxifen effect is favourable irrespective of the oestrogen status of the tumour.

 B tamoxifen cannot suppress carcinoma in the opposite breast.

 C chemotherapy is confined to postmenopausal women.

 D bromocriptine is appropriate.

 E aminoglutethimide produces a medical adrenalectomy.

632. On mammography, the features consistent with the presence of carcinoma include

 A increased skin thickness.

 B assymetry.

 C true microcalcification.

 D a lesion with stellate configuration.

 E several dilated ducts.

633. Gynaecomastia is

 A an abnormal enlargement of the female breast.

 B associated with leprosy

 C encountered in patients with Down's syndrome.

 D associated with ovarian cysts.

 E congenital absence of one breast.

Chapter 13

The thorax
The heart and pericardium

634. If the chest is crushed in a motor accident
- **A** the aorta can be ruptured.
- **B** paradoxical movement is likely to occur.
- **C** early treatment is directed at improving ventilation.
- **D** morphine must not be given.
- **E** a minitracheostomy is contraindicated.

635. Measures taken for the treatment of 'stove-in' chest wall include
- **A** endotracheal intubation
- **B** positive pressure ventilation.
- **C** tracheostomy.
- **D** fixing the rib fractures with stainless steel wire.
- **E** thoracoplasty.

636. Flail chest injury
- **A** occurs when several adjacent ribs are fractured in two places.
- **B** results in paradoxical movement.
- **C** causes a left to right shunt.
- **D** requires endotracheal intubation in severe cases.
- **E** is in itself not an indication for thoracotomy.

637. Isolated rib fractures are characteristically
- **A** painful.
- **B** shown clearly on x-ray.
- **C** associated with Paget's disease of bone.
- **D** a complication of whooping cough.
- **E** not due to direct violence.

638. The management of a haemothorax includes
- **A** apicolysis.
- **B** pleurodesis.
- **C** decortication.
- **D** aspiration.
- **E** thoracotomy.

639. **With traumatic diaphragmatic hernia**
A the diaphragm can be ruptured without an external wound.
B the dome is usually torn in crush injuries.
C a hernia of intestines into the chest follows.
D there is a large hernial sac which becomes adherent to the lungs.
E strangulation does not occur.

640. **The indications for thoracotomy following blunt thoracic trauma include**
A continued brisk bleeding >100 ml/15 min from an intercostal chest drain.
B persistent bleeding >200 ml/h from the drain.
C rupture of the diaphragm.
D fractured sternum.
E cardiac tamponade.

641. **In chest trauma, cardiac injury is suspected when the clinical features include**
A periorbital oedema.
B puffiness of the face.
C subcutaneous emphysema.
D bradycardia.
E muffled heart sounds.

642. **Clinical features associated with cardiac tamponade include**
A raised systolic blood pressure.
B bradycardia.
C Corrigen's pulse.
D faint heart sounds.
E high JVP.

643. **Benign tumours of the ribs include**
A chondroma.
B neurofibroma.
C glomus tumour.
D lipoid granuloma.
E Ewing's tumour.

644. **Benign tumours of the lung include**
A lipoma.
B hamartoma.
C carcinoid adenoma.
D mesothelioma.
E sarcoidosis.

645. **Malignant tumours of the bronchus and lung include**
   A   hamartoma.
   B   carcinoid.
   C   cylindroma.
   D   teratoma.
   E   desmoid tumour.

646. **The histological types of carcinoma of the bronchus include those which are**
   A   round-celled.
   B   squamous-celled.
   C   columnar-celled.
   D   transitional-celled.
   E   oat-celled.

647. **There is a recognised association with carcinoma of the bronchus and**
   A   unresolved 'pneumonia'.
   B   gynaecomastia.
   C   secondary deposits in the brain.
   D   neuropathy without chest symptoms.
   E   Crohn's disease.

648. **Carcinoma of the bronchus can be manifested by**
   A   systemic sclerosis.
   B   epileptiform fits.
   C   gynaecomastia.
   D   hypocalcaemia.
   E   peripheral neuropathy.

649. **Contraindications to radical resection of lung cancer include**
   A   evidence of involvement of the oesophagus.
   B   distant metastases.
   C   generalised arterial disease.
   D   all patients over 65 years.
   E   the presence of lobar collapse.

650. **Anterior mediastinal tumours include**
   A   retrosternal goitre.
   B   teratoma.
   C   neurofibroma.
   D   pleuropericardial cyst.
   E   thymic tumours.

651. Mediastinal cysts include

A spring water cyst.
B 'water lily' cyst.
C foregut cyst.
D pleuropericardial cyst.
E lung cyst.

652. Pleural fluid

A is secreted at the rate of 1 l per day.
B is mainly absorbed by the pleural lymphatics.
C if containing an excess of 30 g protein per litre is an effusion.
D if containing less than 30 g protein per litre is a transudate.
E in cirrhosis of the liver is a transudate.

653. Of the features associated with mesothelioma

A fibrous plaques overlying the pleura are pathognomic.
B pleural effusion is characteristically bilateral.
C night sweats occur.
D lung compression occurs.
E there is commonly a polymorphism of cell types.

654. A pneumothorax

A is the presence of air between the pleura and the rib cage.
B can be spontaneous.
C has the physical signs of a hyperresonant percussion note with absent breath sounds.
D can be recurrent.
E does not cause mediastinal shift.

655. An empyema thoracis

A can occur during staphylococcal pneumonia.
B is preceded usually by a serous effusion.
C if due to pneumococcal infection contains a great deal of fibrin.
D should be drained immediately by rib resection and underwater seal drain.
E is a lung abscess.

656. The management of acute empyema with thin pus includes

A aspiration.
B rib resection.
C decortication.
D tracheostomy.
E Monaldi drainage.

657. **A lung abscess is**
   A   caused by the patient swallowing a tooth after extraction.
   B   commonly due to aspiration pneumonia.
   C   treated by a combination of chemotherapy and lobectomy.
   D   a cause of cerebral abscess.
   E   not associated with malignancy.

658. **Cysts of the lung include those that are**
   A   developmental.
   B   emphysematous.
   C   cysticercotic.
   D   apoplectic.
   E   pseudocysts.

659. **Among the causes and treatment of pulmonary oedema is**
   A   inhalation of phosgene.
   B   fat embolism.
   C   influenzal pneumonia.
   D   the use of intramuscular morphine.
   E   the use of frusemide.

660. **Clinical associations with Boeck's sarcoidosis include**
   A   acquired immune dysfunction.
   B   erythema nodosum.
   C   pulmonary infiltration followed by hilar adenopathy.
   D   secondary infections.
   E   enlarged parotids.

661. **Pulmonary embolism is a condition that characteristically**
   A   is limited to surgical practice.
   B   follows superficial thrombophlebitis.
   C   is a paradoxical embolism.
   D   causes dry gangrene.
   E   is uncommon in equatorial countries.

662. **In a patient with eventration of the diaphragm**
   A   a hiatus hernia is present.
   B   symptoms are uncommon.
   C   volvulus of the stomach may occur.
   D   there is a defect between the sternal and costal attachments.
   E   bowel sounds are heard in the chest.

663. **The anatomical segments of the left lung include the**
A anterior upper.
B superior lingular.
C azygos.
D medial (cardiac).
E lateral basal.

664. **Features associated with mitral stenosis include**
A splinter haemorrhages.
B haematemesis.
C ascites.
D high blood pressure.
E warm vasodilated extremities.

665. **Mitral valvotomy for mitral stenosis**
A is best performed between the ages of 20 and 25 years.
B should be considered when the symptoms are aggravated by pregnancy.
C is not indicated in persistent congestive heart failure.
D gives good results when the mitral valve is immobile.
E is only performed through the left atrium.

666. **With mitral regurgitation**
A even mild degrees cause disability.
B a pansystolic murmur can be heard over the apex.
C papillary muscle rupture can occur acutely.
D an acute onset can lead to acute pulmonary oedema.
E the left ventricle is reduced in size.

667. **Aortic valve stenosis**
A is a cause of sudden death.
B if bicuspid is congenital.
C is associated with a slow rising pulse.
D with a systolic gradient of over 60 mmHg is an indication for valve replacement.
E can be part of Marfan's syndrome.

668. **Clinical associations of infective endocarditis include**
A staphylococcal infections.
B dental treatment.
C peripheal emboli.
D Reiter's syndrome.
E splenomegaly.

669. **The components of Fallot's tetralogy include**
A   an overriding aorta.
B   left ventricular hypertrophy.
C   a persistent ductus.
D   pulmonary tract stenosis.
E   an ASD.

670. **The clinical features of coarctation of the aorta include**
A   headaches.
B   well-developed shoulders compared with the pelvis.
C   Corrigan's pulse.
D   intermittent claudication.
E   warm vasodilated extremities.

671. **In a patient with persistent ductus arteriosus**
A   the pressure in the aorta is higher than in the pulmonary artery.
B   the ductus connects with the right pulmonary artery.
C   as much as 10–20l of blood per minute can flow through.
D   there is a water-hammer pulse.
E   the patient is characteristically adult.

672. **An atrial septal defect**
A   causes overfilling of the left side of the heart.
B   produces a pulmonary systolic murmur.
C   may cause little disability in childhood.
D   can be closed by direct suture under direct vision.
E   is a factor in paradoxical embolism.

673. **Ventricular septal defect**
A   is part of Fallot's tetralogy.
B   causes overfilling of the right heart.
C   is the rarest of congenital cardiac anomalies.
D   results in 50% mortality in the first few months of life.
E   can be multiple.

674. **A ventricular septal defect**
A   is characteristically a single defect.
B   cannot close spontaneously.
C   is associated with infective endocarditis.
D   can be approached surgically through the tricuspid valve.
E   characteristically causes a water-hammer pulse.

675. **If an aortocoronary bypass graft is performed**
   A   the main indication is angina that cannot be controlled by medical means.
   B   coronary arteriography must show a blocked or stenosed coronary artery with a normal vessel beyond.
   C   lengths of femoral vein are used to bypass a narrowed artery.
   D   80–90% can obtain relief from angina.
   E   more than one graft may be required.

676. **Aneurysms of the thoracic aorta have a recognised clinical association with**
   A   Horner's syndrome.
   B   Marfan's syndrome.
   C   atherosclerosis.
   D   ankylosing spondylitis.
   E   paraplegia.

677. **There is a recognised association between cardiac tamponade and**
   A   low systolic blood pressure.
   B   pulsus paradox.
   C   positive Kussmal sign.
   D   central venous catheterisation.
   E   aortic dissection.

678. **Conditions potentially suitable for heart and lung transplantation include**
   A   Cartagena's syndrome.
   B   cystic fibrosis.
   C   bronchial carcinoma invading the pericardium.
   D   fibrosing alveolitis.
   E   toxoplasmosis.

679. **Absolute contraindications to heart transplantation include**
   A   active duodenal ulceration.
   B   malignancy.
   C   alcohol abuse.
   D   HIV positive.
   E   irreversible pulmonary hypertension.

680. **The ideal criteria for a donor heart include**
   A   no evidence of active infection.
   B   no palpable coronary heart disease.
   C   no increased requirements for proton pump inhibitors.
   D   age up to 60 years for a male donor.
   E   ABO compatibility.

681. **Factors recognised to precipitate cardiac arrest include**
   A   hypoxia.
   B   diphtheritic infection.
   C   use of inotropic drugs.
   D   steroids.
   E   iliofemoral embolus.

682. **The immediate treatment of cardiac arrest includes**
   A   intubation.
   B   putting up an i.v. drip.
   C   adrenaline 1 mg iv.
   D   the Holger-Nielsen procedure.
   E   open cardiac massage.

Chapter 14

Anastomoses
The oesophagus
The stomach and duodenum

683. **Factors that are advantageous in the normal healing of intestinal anastomoses include**
   A irradiation.
   B corticosteroid therapy.
   C antibiotic therapy.
   D starch peritonitis.
   E no tension.

684. **In oesophageal anastomoses**
   A horizontal mattress sutures have less tendency to cut through than vertical mattress sutures.
   B the cervical oesophagus can be anastomosed to the stomach.
   C the abdominal oesophagus can be anastomosed to the jejunum by means of a circular stapling device.
   D a Roux-en-Y procedure is contraindicated.
   E a Sengstaken tube can be used to hold an anastomosis in position.

685. **With biliary and pancreatic duct anastomoses acceptable procedures include**
   A Roux-en-Y.
   B using one-layer braided sutures on the biliary tree.
   C an associated gastrojejunostomy in a case of carcinoma of the pancreas.
   D splinting pancreatic duct anastomoses to the jejunum.
   E saphenous vein grafting.

686. **Absorbable suture materials include**
   A polyamide.
   B polymers of glycolide.
   C homopolymer of polydioxanone.
   D polypropylene.
   E collagen.

687. **The complications of an intestinal anastomosis include**
A   haemorrhage.
B   diverticular formation.
C   stenosis.
D   atresia.
E   intussusception.

688. **Lesions recognised to occur at the level of the cricopharyngeal constriction of the oesophagus include**
A   cardiospasm.
B   scleroderma.
C   webs.
D   carcinoma.
E   traction diverticulum.

689. **The sphincter at the lower end of the oesophagus**
A   can be demonstrated anatomically and by histology.
B   serves to prevent reflux of bile.
C   is influenced by smoking.
D   is innervated by the phrenic nerve.
E   loses tone in the presence of loss of lower oesophageal peristaltic activity.

690. **Tracheo-oesophageal fistula is**
A   normally found to be present with atresia.
B   a type of dysphagia lusoria.
C   most frequently present when the lower oesophagus is absent.
D   confirmed necessarily by a barium emulsion swallow.
E   featured by the pouring of saliva from the mouth.

691. **Oesophageal injury**
A   includes that which is by instrumental damage through Killian's dehiscence above the cricopharyngeal sphincter.
B   when due to crushing by an oesophagoscope against an osteoarthritic spine is a component of Boerhaave's syndrome.
C   requires investigation by a barium swallow.
D   requires operative intervention in all cases.
E   symptoms following swallowing corrosives is part of the Mallory-Weiss syndrome.

692. Dysphagia is
   A   the term used only to describe pain on swallowing.
   B   oropharyngeal as well as oesophageal.
   C   only caused by solids.
   D   characteristically vague in its appreciation by the patient.
   E   always present in a patient with hiatus hernia.

693. Clinical associations with oesophagitis include
   A   scalds.
   B   acid reflux.
   C   alkaline reflux.
   D   anaemia.
   E   hiatus hernia.

694. The features of oesophagitis include
   A   the early appearance of dysphagia to fluids before solids.
   B   the presence of occult blood.
   C   heartburn worse when sleeping on the left side.
   D   anginal pain.
   E   white areas of desquamating epithelium on oesophagoscopy.

695. Recognised associations of a hiatus hernia include
   A   eventration of the diaphragm.
   B   infants.
   C   underweight patients.
   D   pneumonitis.
   E   anaemia.

696. Sliding hiatus hernia
   A   is related to scleroderma.
   B   is part of Saint's triad.
   C   accounts for 20% of cases of hiatus hernia.
   D   is the cause of 'congenital short oesophagus'.
   E   is a component of eventration of the diaphragm.

697. There is a recognised association between
   A   hiatus hernia and gallstones.
   B   smoking and Buerger's disease.
   C   melanosis coli and purgatives.
   D   acanthosis nigricans and rodent ulcer.
   E   Paget's disease of the nipple and psoriasis.

698. **Hiatus hernia should be operated upon**
  A   as soon as one course of medical treatment has failed.
  B   if there is significant oesophagitis.
  C   if the hernia is paraoesophageal.
  D   by employing the Nissen fundoplication only.
  E   when it is diagnosed.

699. **Plummer-Vinson syndrome is associated with**
  A   eukonychia.
  B   postcricoid webs.
  C   splenic enlargement.
  D   hepatomegaly.
  E   being a premalignant condition.

700. **Radiological features characteristic of achalasia of the cardia include**
  A   lack of gas bubble in the stomach.
  B   subdiaphragmatic gas shadows.
  C   sigmoid oesophagus.
  D   rat-tailed appearance.
  E   hypersensitivity peristalsis to acetylcholine.

701. **Recognised clinical associations of achalasia of the cardia include**
  A   bronchopneumonia.
  B   food regurgitation.
  C   vitamin B_1 deficiency.
  D   carcinoma of the cardia.
  E   trypanosomiasis.

702. **Scleroderma of the oesophagus is associated with**
  A   acrosclerosis
  B   corkscrew oesophagus.
  C   hiatus hernia.
  D   Peutz-Jeghers syndrome.
  E   proton pump inhibition.

703. **Operations appropriate to stricture of the lower end of the oesophagus include**
  A   regular dilatation
  B   two-thirds Polyá gastrectomy
  C   vagotomy and pyloroplasty.
  D   Thal's patch.
  E   Heller's operation.

704. **In carcinoma of the oesophagus**
   A   50% of the lesions involve the middle third.
   B   about 30% of the patients are women.
   C   from the beginning there is dysphagia to liquids as well as solids.
   D   spread by the blood stream is exceptional.
   E   the cells are oat cells.

705. **In a patient with carcinoma of the midoesophagus**
   A   the lesion is rarely columnar-celled.
   B   lymphatic metastases mainly occur in a downward direction.
   C   regurgitation is common.
   D   radiotherapy is inappropriate.
   E   the surgical results are recognised to be good.

706. **The principles of treatment for oesophageal carcinoma include the use of**
   A   gastrostomy.
   B   radiotherapy for columnar cell lesions.
   C   laser ablation for curative resection.
   D   fine-bore nasogastric feeding.
   E   a Souttar tube.

707. **The gastroduodenal artery is a branch of the**
   A   coeliac axis.
   B   hepatic artery.
   C   superior mesenteric artery.
   D   gastroepiploic artery.
   E   splenic artery.

708. **Of the innervation of the stomach**
   A   the nerves of Auerbach are sympathetic.
   B   parasympathetic nerves include the myenteric plexus of Meissner.
   C   the sympathetic supply comes from the coeliac plexus.
   D   the anterior left vagus supplies fibres to the cardia.
   E   the posterior right vagus forms a plexus on the anterior surface of the stomach.

709. **Gastric mucus**
  A   is produced by the parietal cells.
  B   has a pH of 5.2 to 6.5.
  C   has considerable buffering capacity.
  D   protects the alkaline gastric mucosa.
  E   is composed of glycoprotein.

710. **Gastrin**
  A   is released in response to mechanical distension of the antrum.
  B   is released by the G-cells and reaches the parietal cell by the local splanchnic circulation.
  C   is inhibited when the intragastric pH falls below 3.
  D   release stimulates gastric motor activity by a slight increase in slow wave frequency and a marked increase in associated contractile activity.
  E   is neutralised by oral antacids.

711. **Tests of gastric function now considered acceptable include**
  A   the test meal.
  B   'chew and spit' test.
  C   insulin.
  D   peak acid output.
  E   gastrin assay.

712. **The pillars of the diagnosis of hypertrophic pyloric stenosis of infants rests on**
  A   bile-stained vomit.
  B   diarrhoea.
  C   visible peristalsis.
  D   loss of weight.
  E   presence of a lump.

713. **Concerning operations for hypertrophic pyloric stenosis of infants**
  A   Heller's operation is to be preferred.
  B   perforation of the duodenum at operation is fatal.
  C   hypothermia is a useful adjunct to the operation.
  D   in cases complicated by infection of the mouth, operation should take second place to medical treatment.
  E   breast-fed babies are likely to do better than bottle-fed babies because gastroenteritis is a real problem.

714. **Acute peptic ulcers**
   A   can occur anywhere in the stomach.
   B   seldom invade the muscle layer.
   C   present with haemorrhage.
   D   are rarely multiple.
   E   are associated with ingestion of NSAIDS.

715. **A chronic duodenal ulcer is associated with**
   A   blood group B.
   B   non-β cell tumour.
   C   smoking.
   D   *Helicobacter pylorii* infection.
   E   alkaline gastric mucosa.

716. **A chronic gastric ulcer is**
   A   more common in men than in women.
   B   not associated with smoking.
   C   if a giant ulcer likely to be malignant.
   D   usually situated on the greater curvature of the stomach.
   E   a cause of hour-glass stomach.

717. **The management of chronic peptic ulcers includes**
   A   endoscopic biopsy.
   B   testing for the presence of *Helicobacter pylorii*.
   C   the use of H_2 receptor blockade.
   D   proton pump inhibition.
   E   Bilroth II gastrectomy.

718. **The conservative management of an acute exacerbation of a peptic ulcer includes**
   A   no smoking.
   B   bed rest.
   C   regular meals.
   D   NSAIDs for pain.
   E   sucralfate.

719. **In general the features associated with a duodenal ulcer include**
   A   pain soon after eating but not when lying down.
   B   considerable vomiting.
   C   anorexia nervosa.
   D   heartburn.
   E   well-marked periodicity.

720. **Operation for duodenal ulceration**
   A   gives the best results if performed early in the disease.
   B   is indicated for hour-glass deformity.
   C   carries risks of operation that far outweigh the risks of having an ulcer for 10 years.
   D   includes Bilroth I gastrectomy.
   E   necessarily implies removal of the ulcer.

721. **If a man has had a truncal vagotomy for a duodenal ulcer**
   A   he is often troubled by obstinate constipation.
   B   he tends to get 'blown up' with wind.
   C   a gastric ulcer is a complication.
   D   he tends to suffer from calcium deficiency.
   E   he is very likely to suffer from a bolus obstruction.

722. **If a patient has a partial gastrectomy**
   A   diarrhoea is common, episodic and troublesome.
   B   previous tuberculous disease may be reactivated.
   C   carcinoma of the stomach may occur in the gastric remnant.
   D   bilious vomiting is intermittent rather than with every meal.
   E   megaloblastic anaemia is common and appears about a year after the operation.

723. **In a patient with a perforated peptic ulcer**
   A   if it is a gastric ulcer it could well be malignant.
   B   morphine or other analgesics must not be given until written permission for operation has been obtained.
   C   it is best to perform a gastroscopy before deciding to operate.
   D   the perforation looks oedematous and punched-out.
   E   it is necessary to drain the subhepatic space and the pelvis.

724. **A patient just admitted and being treated conservatively for a bleeding duodenal ulcer is**
   A   allowed to go to the toilet.
   B   given morphine 15 mg i.m. regularly.
   C   given a rapid blood transfusion.
   D   allowed nothing by mouth.
   E   given a small enema to see if he has melaena.

725. **The recognised complications of a duodenal ulcer include**
    A   pyloric stenosis.
    B   penetration.
    C   carcinoma.
    D   hour-glass stomach.
    E   leather bottle stomach.

726. **An hour-glass stomach**
    A   occurs predominantly in men.
    B   is a feature of pyloric stenosis.
    C   is effectively treated by a Bilroth I gastrectomy.
    D   is accompanied by a great loss of weight.
    E   is characteristic of carcinoma of the stomach.

727. **An anastomotic ulcer following operations for duodenal ulcer**
    A   is most likely after a Polyá gastrectomy.
    B   is usually in the mesenteric side of the jejunum.
    C   can contain catgut used in the previous operation.
    D   causes pain that is usually felt in the right hypochondrium and
        travels down the right side of the abdomen.
    E   causes pain that is not relieved by antacids or milk.

728. **Pyloric stenosis**
    A   can be due to a carcinoma at or near the pylorus.
    B   is due to cicatrisation from a duodenal or pyloric gastric ulcer.
    C   classically occurs in men with a long history of ulcer symptoms.
    D   causes hyponatraemia.
    E   occurs in children.

729. **Specific complications of gastroenterostomy include**
    A   duodenal fistula.
    B   pancreatitis.
    C   gastrocolic fistula.
    D   cholangitis.
    E   polycythaemia.

730. **Premalignant risk factors associated with the incidence of carcinoma
    of the stomach include**
    A   polycythaemia.
    B   post-truncal vagotomy stomach.
    C   drinking neat spirits.
    D   Crohn's disease.
    E   excessive ingestion of smoked food.

731. **Recognised associations with carcinoma of the stomach include**
A   blood group O.
B   Troisier's sign.
C   linitis plastica.
D   Krukenberg's tumours.
E   volvulus of the stomach.

732. **In the stomach there is a recognised association with malignant change and**
A   duodenal ulcer.
B   the diameter of a gastric ulcer.
C   the presence of achlorhydria.
D   the growth of cells at the edge of a gastric ulcer that separate the muscularis from the muscularis mucosae.
E   any epithelial downgrowth at the edge of a gastric ulcer.

733. **Carcinoma of the stomach**
A   is a squamous cell tumour.
B   gives a negative test for occult blood.
C   causes a lowered sedimentation rate.
D   is associated with achlorhydria or hypochlorhydria.
E   characteristically begins as a benign gastric ulcer.

734. **In the condition called leather bottle stomach**
A   there is a proliferation of fibrous tissue in the submucosa.
B   the mucous membrane is indurated and hypertrophic.
C   lymph nodes tend not to be affected at an early stage.
D   Crohn's disease is the differential diagnosis.
E   gastrectomy is likely to be curative.

735. **The prognosis following resection of carcinoma of the stomach is specifically determined by**
A   the extent of stomach removed.
B   the margin of apparently healthy stomach removed above the growth.
C   a short clinical history.
D   the histology of the growth.
E   the sex of the patient.

736. Regarding foreign bodies in the stomach
  A if a patient has several foreign bodies in the stomach it is likely that these have been swallowed on purpose.
  B they should always be removed promptly by operation.
  C they tend to be radiolucent.
  D fibreoptic gastroscopy should replace operations for their removal.
  E if they pass round into the jejunum it is likely that they will impact in the ileum.

737. Postoperative acute dilatation of the stomach is suggested by the appearance of
  A hiccups
  B effortless vomit.
  C dark watery vomit.
  D considerable flatus.
  E shock.

738. Volvulus of the stomach is associated with
  A tricobezoar.
  B eventration of the diaphragm.
  C duodenal ileus.
  D acute dilatation of the stomach.
  E inversion of the greater curvature of the stomach.

739. A duodenal fistula
  A is a complication of trauma to the duodenum.
  B is a complication of gastrostomy.
  C can follow a right hemicolectomy.
  D causes excoriation of the skin.
  E requires immediate operation to prevent dehydration and hypoproteinaemia.

740. A gastrocolic fistula characteristically
  A presents by the vomiting of faeces.
  B is a cause of steatorrhoea.
  C does not involve the function of the small intestine.
  D causes all the gastric contents to pass directly into the colon.
  E is caused by gall-stones.

Chapter 15

The liver
The spleen
The gall bladder and bile ducts
The pancreas

741. Liver function tests in common usage include those that measure the
A   creatinine kinase.
B   serum acid phosphatase activity.
C   serum γ-glutamyl transferase activity.
D   blood cholesterol.
E   serum albumin level.

742. Liver biopsy can be
A   performed safely on any person.
B   performed by using a Menghini needle.
C   reliable as a means of detecting tumours.
D   carried out via the epigastrium.
E   profitably combined with peritoneoscopy.

743. The occurrence of portosystemic encephalopathy is associated with
A   ammonia.
B   a portosystemic shunt.
C   hyponatraemia.
D   parkinsonism.
E   cogwheel rigidity.

744. Operative measures conducive to the successful management of traumatic rupture of the liver include
A   doing the minimum necessary to control the bleeding.
B   the use of packing.
C   coeliac axis ligation.
D   major hepatic resection.
E   checking the spleen.

745. Cholangitis is
A   thrombophlebitis of small hepatic veins.
B   pyelophlebitis.
C   inflammation of the bile ducts.
D   a form of angina.
E   associated with gall-stones.

746. **Idiopathic liver abscess is associated with**
  A   malnutrition.
  B   pleural effusion
  C   cryptogenicity.
  D   marked leucocytosis.
  E   amoebiasis.

747. **Amoebic abscess of the liver**
  A   is caused by *Entamoeba coli.*
  B   contains chocolate- or pink-coloured pus.
  C   can become encapsulated.
  D   has pus that is nearly always sterile.
  E   is better treated by the use of drainage tubes than by repeated aspiration.

748. **In chronic abscesses of the liver**
  A   no cause can be found in half the cases.
  B   the presence of leucocytosis is helpful in making the diagnosis.
  C   ultrasound will localise the abscess.
  D   the condition is fatal unless drained by laparotomy.
  E   if amoebic in origin should be drained by means of a drainage tube through the abdominal wall.

749. **In hydatid disease due to echinococcal infestation**
  A   the worm ova are shed by dogs.
  B   the worm contains a body comprised of one segment.
  C   the ovum bears two hooklets.
  D   the condition does not occur where there are no sheep.
  E   a hydatid cyst is composed of two layers.

750. **With a hydatid cyst**
  A   the endocyst secretes the hydatid fluid.
  B   the scolices develop within the brood capsules.
  C   the pseudocyst looks like a colourless balloon filled with water.
  D   calcification means deterioration in the host.
  E   damage to the laminated membrane encourages the formation of daughter cysts.

751. **Clinical associations of cirrhosis of the liver include**
  A   gynaecomastia.
  B   testicular atrophy.
  C   koilonychia.
  D   Dupuytren's contracture.
  E   achalasia of the cardia.

752. The causes of cirrhosis of the liver in the adult include

A   *Entamoeba histolytica* infestation.
B   ulcerative colitis.
C   malaria.
D   schistosomiasis.
E   nutritional deficiency.

753. Suitable methods employed to control bleeding from oesophageal varices include

A   splenectomy
B   vasopressin i.v.
C   passing a Sengstaken tube.
D   passing a Fogarty catheter.
E   sclerotherapy.

754. Oesophageal varices

A   are restricted to the oesophagus.
B   can be demonstrated by splenic-portography.
C   can always be demonstrated by oesophagoscopy.
D   can be treated by injection.
E   relate to cirrhosis of the liver.

755. Portasystemic shunting operations

A   should not be performed if the patient is significantly jaundiced.
B   should not be performed if the patient's serum albumin is more than 30 g/l (3 g/100 ml).
C   should be reserved for patients who are bleeding from varices.
D   are avoided in the presence of ascites.
E   are needed to prevent bleeding from oesophageal varices before it ever happens.

756. Budd-Chiari syndrome is associated with

A   polycythaemia.
B   hepatolenticular degeneration.
C   the use of hormones for infertility.
D   haemochromatosis.
E   congenital web in the IVC.

150

757. **Of the benign tumours of the liver, the**
   A hepatoadenoma is associated with the use of oral contraceptives.
   B hepatoadenoma is premalignant.
   C cholangioadenoma is premalignant.
   D haemangioma is usually a port wine stain.
   E haemangioma can be of a malignant type.

758. **Primary carcinoma of the liver**
   A tends to occur in children and older people.
   B causes a Pel-Ebstein type of fever.
   C causes the CEA level in the plasma to be raised.
   D cannot be diagnosed by CT scanning.
   E is associated with ascites in about 40% of patients at the time of first examination.

759. **Liver metastases are**
   A umbilicated.
   B confidently diagnosed by palpation at laparotomy.
   C treated by enucleation.
   D associated with primary melanoma in the eye.
   E a cause of pyrexia.

760. **The spleen**
   A provides 500 ml of blood to add to the circulation in case of haemorrhage.
   B destroys effete erythrocytes.
   C is a platelet reservoir.
   D forms erythrocytes and lymphocytes.
   E causes spherocytosis.

761. **The recognised functions of the spleen include**
   A production of VIP.
   B antibody production.
   C platelet phagocytosis.
   D production of calcitonin.
   E erythropoiesis in myelofibrosis.

762. **The clinical features of a ruptured spleen include**
   A abdominal distension.
   B ladder pattern.
   C Boas's sign.
   D guarding.
   E sighing respiration.

763. **Recognised radiological features of a ruptured spleen include**
   A   subdiaphragmatic gas shadows.
   B   elevation of the left side of the diaphragm.
   C   obliteration of the psoas shadow.
   D   eventration of the diaphragm.
   E   free fluid between gas-filled coils of intestine.

764. **Idiopathic thrombocytopenic purpura is**
   A   a cause of intussusception.
   B   a cause of haematuria.
   C   manifests as large areas of bruising.
   D   confirmed by the appearance of petechiae after a sphyg-
        momanometer cuff is inflated above the systolic pressure for 10
        minutes.
   E   due to vitamin B deficiency.

765. **In the haemolytic anaemias**
   A   spherocytosis is due to abnormal immunological responses.
   B   chronic ulcers of the legs occur in congenital haemolytic
        anaemia.
   C   the liver may be palpable.
   D   the patients tend to suffer from gall-stones.
   E   ACTH is the general mainspring of treatment.

766. **Purpura occurs characteristically in a patient who has**
   A   a thrombocytopathy.
   B   port wine staining.
   C   venous gangrene.
   D   phlegmasia caerulea dolens.
   E   septicaemia.

767. **A patient with idiopathic thrombocytopenic purpura characteristically**
   A   is more likely to get purpuric lesions in the dependent areas.
   B   has Felty's syndrome.
   C   tends to respond to steroid therapy.
   D   is rarely helped in the control of the bleeding tendency by
        splenectomy.
   E   can suffer intracranial haemorrhage.

152

768. **Acquired autoimmune haemolytic anaemia**
   A   can be due to a drug reaction.
   B   is associated with systemic lupus erythematosus.
   C   is associated with damage to the surface of the red cell.
   D   is a cause of cystine stones.
   E   is a contraindication to splenectomy.

769. **Features characteristic of sickle-cell disease include**
   A   replacement of HbS by HbA.
   B   crystallisation of the Hb molecule when blood O_2 tension increases.
   C   bone pain.
   D   abdominal pain.
   E   autosplenectomy.

770. **Tropical splenomegaly**
   A   follows amoebic dysentery.
   B   can be caused by malaria.
   C   is caused by Chlamydia trachomatis.
   D   causes thrombocytopenia.
   E   is often benefited by splenectomy.

771. **Cysts of the spleen include the**
   A   dermoid.
   B   choledochal.
   C   aneurysmal bone.
   D   traumatic.
   E   lymphatic.

772. **The effects of splenectomy include**
   A   changes in the bone marrow.
   B   hypertrophy of any splenunculi.
   C   eosinophilia.
   D   leucopenia.
   E   immunodeficiency.

773. **Essential stages of the elective removal of the spleen include**
   A   a Morris incision.
   B   as the first step to pass a hand round the outer surface of the spleen to avulse adhesions and to divide the posterior layer of the lienorenal ligament.
   C   the lesser sac between stomach, colon and spleen being opened to give access to the splenic vessels.
   D   looking for splenunculi.
   E   wound drainage even if haemostasis is satisfactory.

774. **In the surgical physiology of the biliary system**
   A   the bile on leaving the liver contains 10% bile salts.
   B   the liver excretes bile at a rate of some 40 ml/h.
   C   the gall bladder excretes sodium chloride.
   D   cholecystokinin controls the production of bile salts.
   E   the gall bladder concentrates bile 5–10 times.

775. **Regarding radiological investigations of the biliary tree**
   A   ultrasound is the first choice.
   B   plain x-ray shows up radiolucent gall-stones.
   C   a cholecystogram is performed after breakfast 12 hours following the ingestion of the contrast medium.
   D   cholecystography is valueless if the plasma bilirubin level is over 3 mg/100 ml (51 µmol/l).
   E   the contrast medium contains iodine with an atomic weight of 131.

776. **Peroperative cholangiography**
   A   reveals the presence of gall-stones in the common hepatic duct.
   B   confirms the anatomy of the ducts.
   C   confirms the patency of the duodenal papilla.
   D   confirms the anatomy of the arterial supply to the gall bladder and liver.
   E   has to be performed by the transhepatic route.

777. **Regarding congenital atresia of the bile ducts**
   A   it tends to be caused by neonatal hepatitis.
   B   meconium is clay-coloured at birth.
   C   the mother has hereditary spherocytosis.
   D   operative cholangiography is impossible because of the size of the ducts.
   E   surgery has very little to offer in such cases.

778. **Mixed gall-stones**
    A   contain calcium.
    B   can contain Salmonella.
    C   constitute the majority of gall-stones.
    D   can be faceted.
    E   contain bilirubin.

779. **Recognised constituents and clinical associations of gall-stones include**
    A   protein.
    B   bacteria.
    C   oxalates.
    D   malaria.
    E   acholuric jaundice.

780. **Pure cholesterol stones are**
    A   single.
    B   multiple.
    C   light in weight.
    D   radio-opaque.
    E   at the centre of combination stones.

781. **Gall-stones**
    A   are always the cause of flatulent dyspepsia.
    B   are becoming common in postpartum primipara who were prepregnancy 'Pill' takers.
    C   can be present in the newborn.
    D   cause mucocele of the gall bladder.
    E   can form as primary stones in the common bile duct.

782. **The conservative treatment for acute cholecystitis**
    A   is avoided in typhoidal cholecystitis.
    B   has a higher morbidity than emergency operation.
    C   has a higher mortality than emergency operation.
    D   only results in resolution in 40% of the cases.
    E   is likely to reduce the chances of damage to the common bile ducts at an elective operation compared with an emergency operation.

783. In 15% of patients on whom cholecystectomy has been performed the symptoms for which the operation was performed persist. These could be due to the presence of

A an abscess of the cystic duct remnant.
B a hiatus hernia.
C a motility disorder of the duodenum and choledochal sphincter.
D pancreatitis.
E a stone remaining in the common bile duct.

784. Of the lesions known collectively as the cholecystoses

A the strawberry gall bladder is so called because of the subserous collections of cholesterol.
B polyposis is evident on cholecystography.
C intramural diverticulosis occurs with cholecystitis glandularis proliferans.
D biliary fistula is a recognised complication of cholecystitis glandularis proliferans.
E squamous metaplasia is included as one of these.

785. Cholangitis is

A thrombophlebitis of small hepatic veins.
B pyelophlebitis.
C inflammation of the bile ducts.
D a form of angina.
E associated with gall-stones.

786. In an attack of gall-stone colic, the patient characteristically

A lies still, afraid to move.
B is doubled up.
C may roll on the floor.
D has pain in the tip of the left shoulder.
E has pain across the upper abdomen.

787. Courvoisier's law concerns

A the length of a skin flap in skin grafting.
B ureteric colic.
C obstruction of the common bile duct.
D alveolar gases.
E fibroblastic response.

788. Charcot's biliary triad includes
  A   itching of the skin.
  B   fluctuating jaundice.
  C   recurrent pain.
  D   constant pale stools.
  E   intermittent fever.

789. Gall-stones in the common bile duct are extracted by means of
  A   cholecystostomy.
  B   ERCP.
  C   sphincterotomy (of the duodenal papilla).
  D   cholecystectomy and choledochotomy.
  E   choledochoscopy.

790. A choledochus cyst is
  A   congenital.
  B   parasitic.
  C   more common in males than in females.
  D   lined by squamous epithelium.
  E   a cause of jaundice.

791. Strictures of the common bile duct
  A   are usually due to operative trauma.
  B   are related to ignorance of the anatomical anomalies of the bile ducts.
  C   can be due to sclerosing cholangitis.
  D   present immediately after operation with jaundice.
  E   can be repaired over a T-tube.

792. Choledochoduodenostomy
  A   is an alternative procedure to transduodenal sphincterotomy.
  B   is especially applicable for ductal stones and sludge in the elderly.
  C   is contraindicated if the duct is not more than 1.5 cm in diameter.
  D   necessitates the insertion of a pigtail stent.
  E   is applicable for the treatment of asiatic cholangiohepatitis.

793. Carcinoma of the gall bladder
  A   is either an extension of carcinoma of the pancreas or a cholangiocarcinoma.
  B   usually starts in the cystic duct and neck of the gall bladder.
  C   can be a squamous cell carcinoma.
  D   is more common in women than in men.
  E   uncommonly metastasises.

794. Carcinoma of the gall bladder
  A   accounts for 10% of all malignant neoplasms.
  B   is associated with the presence of gall-stones in 90% of cases.
  C   may begin by squamous metaplasia.
  D   carries a dismal prognosis (2% surviving five years).
  E   remains confined to the gall bladder.

795. In the surgical anatomy of the pancreas the
  A   head overlies the first lumbar vertebra.
  B   accessory duct enters the second part of the duodenum.
  C   superior mesenteric vessels pass behind the uncinate process.
  D   superior mesenteric artery lies to the right of the superior mesenteric vein.
  E   superior mesenteric vein joins the portal vein behind the head of the pancreas.

796. The pancreatic secretion
  A   of bicarbonate rich fluid is increased by pancreozymin.
  B   of enzymes is increased by secretin.
  C   of bicarbonate comes from acinar cells.
  D   of enzymes comes from ductal cells.
  E   is inhibited by glucagon.

797. Beside the pancreas, amylases are to be found in the
  A   salivary glands.
  B   liver.
  C   adrenals.
  D   lactating breast.
  E   the fallopian tubes.

798. **Cystic fibrosis of the pancreas**
   A   accompanies congenital cystic disease of the kidneys and liver.
   B   is a manifestation of a hereditary congenital abnormality of mucus secretion.
   C   causes intestinal obstruction.
   D   encourages staphylococcal infections.
   E   causes excessive loss of sodium chloride in the sweat.

799. **The Marseilles classification of pancreatitis includes**
   A   relapsing acute pancreatitis.
   B   idiopathic pancreatitis.
   C   chronic pancreatitis.
   D   relapsing chronic pancreatitis.
   E   alcoholic pancreatitis.

800. **There is a recognised association between acute pancreatitis and**
   A   fat necrosis.
   B   cholelithiasis.
   C   mumps.
   D   leucopenia.
   E   sulphaemoglobinaemia.

801. **If a patient is believed to have acute pancreatitis**
   A   laparotomy is essential if there is any doubt about the diagnosis.
   B   morphine in the treatment of the pain should be used in conjunction with pethidine (demerol or demerol hydrochloride).
   C   intravenous fluids increase the oedema of the pancreas.
   D   gall-stones are present in at least 30% of patients.
   E   a pseudocyst can occur later.

802. **Grey Turner's sign in acute pancreatitis is a**
   A   discoloration in the loins.
   B   shifting dullness over the spleen.
   C   discoloration around the umbilicus.
   D   fluid level seen on x-ray in the first loop of the jejunum.
   E   soreness of the skin beside the vertebral border of the right scapula.

803. **The treatment of acute pancreatitis**
   A   should be conservative if there is any doubt about the diagnosis.
   B   includes the use of atropine or propantheline.
   C   includes calcium gluconate intravenously.
   D   includes large doses of antibiotics.
   E   is immediate laparotomy and pancreatectomy.

804. **Complications of acute pancreatitis include**
   A   'third space' collection.
   B   hypoxia.
   C   hypercalcaemia.
   D   hypertension.
   E   pseudocyst.

805. **If a patient has chronic pancreatitis**
   A   the volume of secretion as a result of the secretinpancreozymin test is reduced.
   B   a needle biopsy to distinguish between it and carcinoma should be performed through the epigastrium.
   C   alcohol is permitted in small quantities.
   D   and pain is severe, chemical sphlanchnicectomy under x-ray television control is applicable.
   E   cholecystojejunostomy with enteroenterostomy is suitable if jaundice is present.

806. **True cysts of the pancreas**
   A   are characteristically more common than pseudocysts.
   B   present as a solid swelling.
   C   can be attributed to *Echinococcus taenia*.
   D   if in the head, are treated by pancreaticoduodenectomy (Whipple's operation).
   E   if in the body, are suitable for cystogastrostomy.

807. **Carcinoma of the pancreas**
   A   occurs mostly in the head of the gland.
   B   is associated with a distended gall bladder.
   C   can cause the passage of 'aluminium' stools.
   D   is not related to diabetes.
   E   causes mucoviscidosis.

808. **Features recognised to be associated with carcinoma of the pancreas include the facts that**
   A   most cases are adenocarcinomas of cell duct origin.
   B   jaundice is synonymous with ampullary carcinoma.
   C   the liver is palpable in 80% of cases.
   D   the gall bladder is distended in 50% of ampullary tumours.
   E   splenic vein thrombosis is an associated feature.

809. **A characteristic of carcinoma of the pancreas is that**
   A   70% of the patients have a periampullary carcinoma.
   B   it is usually a medullary carcinoma.
   C   if occurring in the body and tail it tends to involve the duodeno-jejunal junction.
   D   Troisier's sign is commonly positive.
   E   the patient may present with copious watery bright green vomit.

810. **The presence of carcinoma of the pancreas can be indicated by**
   A   thrombophlebitis migrans.
   B   diabetes.
   C   pancreatic calcinosis.
   D   the ordinary three sign on a barium meal.
   E   the triple response of Lewis.

811. **Useful investigations in patients suspected of suffering from carcinoma of the pancreas include**
   A   hypotonic duodenogram.
   B   pancreatic ultrasound.
   C   ERCP.
   D   gastrin assay.
   E   fasting blood sugar.

812. **A patient with an insulinoma**
   A   has an alpha-cell tumour of the pancreas.
   B   may be in a mental hospital.
   C   displays Saint's triad and this establishes the diagnosis.
   D   has an identifiable hypoglycaemia with fasting up to 72 hours.
   E   is likely to suffer from the Zollinger-Ellison syndrome.

813. Zollinger-Ellison syndrome is associated with
  A antral G-cell hyperplasia.
  B carcinoid tumour.
  C jejunal ulceration.
  D hyperkalaemia.
  E Whipple's triad.

Chapter 16

The peritoneum, omentum, mesentery and retroperitoneum
The intestines
Intestinal obstruction
The appendix

814. Factors favouring diffusion of peritonitis include
A   sudden perforation.
B   drinking some water.
C   giving an enema.
D   sitting the patient up in bed.
E   the use of morphine.

815. Clinical features associated with diffuse peritonitis initially include
A   Hippocratic facies.
B   vomiting.
C   a patient who is afraid to cough.
D   the presence of bowel sounds.
E   hyperpyrexia.

816. In generalised peritonitis
A   the patient rolls around in agony.
B   morphine or pethidine (demerol USP) is useful while the patient is under observation.
C   operation is contraindicated.
D   the pulse rate falls progressively.
E   the cause can be other than performation of the gastrointestinal tract.

817. In a patient with a pelvic abscess
A   pus can accumulate without serious constitutional disturbance.
B   constipation is a characteristic symptom.
C   the abscess feels like a hard apple on rectal examination.
D   the abscess may discharge spontaneously through the rectum.
E   drainage should be achieved by means of a low abdominal laparotomy.

818. **The subphrenic spaces where abscesses occur include the**
   A   midline extraperitoneal.
   B   midline intraperitoneal.
   C   right posterior intraperitoneal.
   D   lesser sac.
   E   left anterior intraperitoneal.

819. **In a patient with a subphrenic abscess**
   A   there is loss of weight.
   B   there can be a pleural effusion.
   C   there is a relative but not absolute leucocytosis.
   D   needling through the ninth intercostal space is performed prior to exposure and opening of a posterior supradiaphragmatic abscess.
   E   a fine bore drainage tube should be left in after opening the abscess.

820. **Prolonged parental antibiotic therapy**
   A   is necessary for subphrenic abscess.
   B   is necessary for ileocaecal actinomycosis.
   C   can cause intestinal obstruction if used for peritonitis.
   D   can mask the general signs of an intra-abdominal abscess.
   E   characteristically causes staphylococcal enterocolitis.

821. **Secondary malignant deposits observed in the peritoneal cavity can be confused with**
   A   peritoneal hydatids.
   B   tuberculous peritonitis.
   C   fat necrosis.
   D   pneumococcal peritonitis.
   E   omental pearls (peritoneal mice).

822. **According to the type, tuberculous peritonitis**
   A   can be confused with peritoneal carcinomatosis.
   B   can cause congenital hydroceles to appear.
   C   can be confused with an ovarian cyst.
   D   if causing obstruction should be treated by anastomosis between an obviously dilated loop and a collapsed loop of intestine.
   E   can present as a cold abscess near the umbilicus.

823. **The causes of ascites includes**
    A   Meigs' syndrome.
    B   endometriosis.
    C   pseudomyxoma peritoneii.
    D   Pick's disease.
    E   Arnold-Chiari malformation.

824. **Regarding paracentesis abdominis**
    A   it may be employed in congestive cardiac failure.
    B   it may be employed for the Arnold-Chiari malformation.
    C   a local anaesthetic is unnecessary.
    D   the fluid should always be drawn off quickly once flow is established.
    E   tapping at regular intervals is satisfactory.

825. **A wound of the mesentery of the small intestine**
    A   causes pneumoperitoneum.
    B   is commonly associated with rupture of the intestine.
    C   if transverse is treated electively by suturing the tear.
    D   should be suspected if there is bruising of the abdominal wall following a car accident, even if seat belts were worn.
    E   requires exteriorisation of the affected coil of intestine.

826. **Recognised clinical features associated with a mesenteric cyst include**
    A   a hard swelling near the umbilicus.
    B   a swelling which moves freely in line with the attachment of the mesentery.
    C   recurrent attacks of abdominal pain.
    D   an acute abdominal catastrophe.
    E   a positive Grey Turner's sign.

827. **The types of mesenteric cyst include**
    A   the dermoid.
    B   the chylolymphatic.
    C   the enterogenous.
    D   a urogenital remnant.
    E   Ormond's disease.

828. **Retroperitoneal tumours include**
    A   ganglioneuroma.
    B   lipoma.
    C   sarcoma.
    D   enterogenous cysts.
    E   desmoid tumours.

829. There is a recognised association between retroperitoneal fibrosis and
  A the injection of haemorrhoids.
  B carcinoid.
  C pulmonary fibrosis.
  D Dupuytren's contracture.
  E sarcoidosis.

830. If a newborn infant is suffering from Hirschsprung's disease
  A the condition becomes apparent about three weeks after birth.
  B the rectum feels empty and grips the examining finger.
  C on withdrawing the examining finger from the anus there may be a short squirt of meconium.
  D the caecum can perforate.
  E total colectomy is necessary.

831. Features relating to angiodysplasia of the colon include
  A haemorrhagic shock.
  B ischaemic colitis.
  C cirsoid aneurysm.
  D vascular degeneration.
  E angiographic 'blush'.

832. Recognised associations with blind-loop syndrome include
  A jejunal diverticula.
  B postvagotomy syndrome.
  C vitamin B6 deficiency.
  D gastrocolic fistula.
  E steatorrhoea.

833. Meckel's diverticulum
  A is present in 20% of the human race.
  B arises from the mesenteric border of the jejunum.
  C may contain heterotopic pancreas.
  D is only present in the male sex.
  E is a diverticulum of the bladder.

834. Diverticular disease is characteristically
  A restricted to the sigmoid colon.
  B associated with gastric ulceration.
  C related to the sites where blood vessels penetrate the bowel wall.
  D precancerous.
  E essentially congenital in origin.

835. **If a woman aged 60 has diverticulitis of the sigmoid colon**
A she is likely to have gall-stones and a hiatus hernia.
B on a barium enema the condition is localised with no relaxation with propanthelin.
C bleeding is often periodic and profuse.
D she is likely to have a vesicovaginal fistula.
E excision of the affected area is unequivocally recommended.

836. **Operations that are suitable for patients with diverticulitis**
A in remission and prepared – a one stage resection.
B if obstructed – a Hartmann procedure.
C if acutely perforated – primary resection and Hartmann.
D in remission – a Paul Mikulicz procedure.
E in remission – a caecostomy.

837. **Complications of ulcerative colitis include**
A neuropathic joints.
B stomatitis.
C iritis.
D renal calculi.
E skin lesions.

838. **Features associated with Crohn's disease include**
A faecal fistula.
B steatorrhoea.
C cholangitis.
D calcified lymph nodes.
E apple core filling defect of a colonic lesion on barium enema.

839. **There is a recognised association between**
A Crohn's disease and fistula in ano.
B fistula in ano and ischiorectal abscess.
C ischiorectal abscess and pilonidal sinus.
D pilonidal sinus and umbilical discharge.
E umbilical discharge and patent urachus.

840. **Intestinal amoebiasis.**
A is unknown in the United Kingdom.
B is due to the effects of *Entamoeba coli*.
C can perforate the caecum.
D causes a carcinoma of the colon.
E causes a liver abscess which contains pus that is said to look like anchovy sauce.

841. **The complications of typhoid infection include**
  A   paralytic ileus.
  B   intestinal haemorrhage.
  C   gall-stone formation.
  D   osteomyelitis.
  E   laryngitis.

842. **A patient with a faecal fistula in the right iliac fossa**
  A   which occurs after appendicectomy, may have actinomycosis.
  B   could be asked to swallow a methylene blue tablet in order to prove the presence of the fistula.
  C   should be treated by an operation for closure of the fistula itself.
  D   should not be given anything by mouth.
  E   will need an ileostomy.

843. **Concerning tumours of the small intestine**
  A   a leiomyoma can cause an intussusception.
  B   brown pigmentation of the oral mucosa is the *sine qua non* of Peutz-Jeghers syndrome.
  C   lymphosarcoma runs a rapid course and is untreatable.
  D   adenocarcinoma does not occur in the jejunum.
  E   a carcinoid tumour of the lower ileum should be resected by a right hemicolectomy.

844. **Of the benign tumours of the large intestine**
  A   adenomatous polyps and villous tumours are synonymous.
  B   villous tumours are associated with acute hyponatraemia.
  C   the hamartomatous polyps are characteristically premalignant.
  D   FAP is associated with chromosome 5.
  E   FAP is associated with desmoids.

845. **There is a recognised association between carcinoma of the caecum and**
  A   anaemia.
  B   appendicitis.
  C   steatorrhoea.
  D   intussusception.
  E   pneumaturia.

846. **Symptoms relating to carcinoma of the sigmoid colon include**
    A   vomiting.
    B   indigestion.
    C   alteration of bowel habit.
    D   abdominal pain.
    E   bleeding per rectum.

847. **Carcinoma of the colon characteristically**
    A   spreads to inguinal lymph nodes
    B   is transitional celled.
    C   presents early when on the right side.
    D   is markedly radiosensitive.
    E   causes anaemia.

848. **Carcinoma of the**
    A   caecum should be treated by caecectomy.
    B   hepatic flexure can involve the right ureter.
    C   transverse colon is best treated if the excision includes the hepatic and the splenic flexure.
    D   splenic flexure is best excised with four inches of transverse and descending colon (above and below).
    E   pelvic colon is resected together with the splenic flexure.

849. **Temporary loop colostomy is**
    A   indicated for ulcerative colitis.
    B   indicated in the treatment of vesicocolic fistula.
    C   usually made with the transverse colon.
    D   opened immediately at the end of the operation.
    E   best closed by extraperitoneal methods.

850. **The complications of colostomies include**
    A   atresia.
    B   stenosis.
    C   prolapse.
    D   necrosis.
    E   desmoid formation.

851. **Features associated with intestinal obstruction include**
    A   aerophagy.
    B   ladder pattern.
    C   toxaemia.
    D   hypovolaemia.
    E   the Arnold-Chiari malformation.

852. **In intestinal obstruction with strangulation**
    A   volvulus is one cause.
    B   the loss of circulating blood volume due to strangulation of several feet of small intestine is considerable.
    C   when vascular obstruction occurs the artery is compressed first.
    D   there is more toxic absorption into the circulation from strangulation in an external hernia than from an internal strangulation.
    E   embolectomy is the rational procedure.

853. **With congenital problems causing acute intestinal obstruction in the newborn**
    A   atresia and stenosis of the duodenum occur with about equal frequency.
    B   supraduodenal atresia is distinguished from oeseophagal atresia by the fact that there is no dribbling of saliva.
    C   meconium ileus is due to ileal atresia.
    D   volvulus of the midgut includes the caecum.
    E   atresia of the ileum may present as a perforation.

854. **Intussusception is related to**
    A   muscoviscidosis.
    B   swollen Peyer's patches.
    C   intestinal volvulus.
    D   a Richter's hernia.
    E   a patent vitello intestinal duct.

855. **Volvulus of the intestines.**
    A   only affects adults.
    B   is not a cause of strangulation.
    C   characteristically follows volvulus of the stomach.
    D   is unknown in India.
    E   is associated with Meig's syndrome.

856. **Bolus obstruction**
    A   can follow eating unripe apples.
    B   is a complication after partial gastrectomy.
    C   can be caused by a gall-stone.
    D   is treated by enemas.
    E   should be investigated by an emergency barium meal.

857. **When faecal impaction occurs it**
 A   causes absolute constipation.
 B   is manifest by the passage of flatus but not faeces.
 C   is suspected when it is reported that an elderly patient has faecal incontinence or diarrhoea.
 D   causes abdominal pain and faeces may be palpable through the abdominal wall.
 E   is likely to require disimpaction with the aid of the fingers or a spoon.

858. **In the management of paralytic ileus**
 A   morphine is strictly contraindicated.
 B   a nasogastric tube should not be spiggotted.
 C   lowering of the serum potassium level is a welcome sign.
 D   daily measurement of the abdominal girth is mandatory.
 E   hunger pains indicate worsening of the problem.

859. **Ischaemic colitis**
 A   usually affects the caecum and ascending colon.
 B   can follow insertion of an aortofemoral prosthesis for an abdominal aneurysm.
 C   can occur in Buerger's disease (thromboangiitis obliterans).
 D   can occur in atheroslerosis.
 E   should be treated by steroids.

860. **Acute obstructive appendicitis**
 A   is the most common type.
 B   can be caused by carcinoma of the caecum.
 C   can occur in a hernia.
 D   can accompany ileocaecal Crohn's disease.
 E   is rare before the age of two years.

861. **Characteristically in acute appendicitis**
 A   the tongue is clean.
 B   rigidity can be absent if the appendix is pelvic in position.
 C   vomiting always precedes pain.
 D   the pain begins in the RIF.
 E   conservative treatment is the rule.

862. The differential diagnosis of acute appendicitis includes

A   pneumonia.
B   cyclical vomiting.
C   acute pyelonephritis.
D   porphyria.
E   Barrett's ulcer.

863. Regarding appendicectomy for acute appendicitis

A   the incision should relate to the position in which the appendix is thought to lie.
B   a Kocher's incision is useful for a pelvic appendix.
C   it is not necessary to bury the stump of the appendix.
D   haemostasis is achieved by diathermy.
E   the peritoneal cavity should be drained.

864. A localised mass in the right iliac fossa, thought to be due to appendicitis, yet with the patient in a satisfactory condition

A   is an indication for immediate appendicectomy.
B   should be treated conservatively with light diet, analgesics and mild intestinal evacuants.
C   should be explored in children
D   should be explored in patients over 65 years.
E   is an indication for long-term oral antibiotics to be started.

Chapter 17

The rectum
The anus and anal canal

865. An immediate relation to the rectum in the female includes the
A   superior rectal artery anteriorly.
B   urethra.
C   posterior vaginal wall posteriorly.
D   levator ani muscle laterally.
E   pouch of Douglas anteriorly.

866. Relations of the rectum in the male include the facts that
A   the prostate is separated anteriorly by Waldeyer's fascia.
B   laterally lies the levator ani.
C   laterally lies the superior rectal artery.
D   posteriorly the coccyx and the last two sacral vertebrae are separated by Denonvillier's fascia.
E   posteriorly lies the obturator internus muscle.

867. Characteristic of the lymphatics of the rectum is that the
A   lymphatic vessels of the submucosa do not connect with the subfascial vessels.
B   drainage is usually upwards.
C   lymph flow can be retrograde.
D   the superior rectal nodes overlie the aortic bifurcation.
E   the middle rectal nodes lie around the internal iliac arteries.

868. Symptoms of rectal disease include
A   spurious diarrhoea.
B   strangury.
C   pruritus.
D   prolapse.
E   hesitancy.

869. Partial prolapse of the rectum
A   occurs in elderly people as well as in children.
B   can occur in whooping cough.
C   is predisposed to by a torn perineum.
D   is characteristically plum-coloured.
E   can be treated successfully by Thiersch's operation.

870. **Complete prolapse of the rectum**
    A   is common in children.
    B   is virtually an intussusception of the rectum upon itself, but there is no intussuscipiens.
    C   when large may contain a pouch of peritoneum containing small intestine.
    D   can be distinguished from rectosigmoid intussusception.
    E   is best excised.

871. **Proctitis is associated with**
    A   proctalgia fugax.
    B   pseudomembranous colitis.
    C   amoebic granuloma.
    D   Crohn's disease.
    E   granuloma inguinale.

872. **The solitary rectal ulcer**
    A   characteristically occurs on the posterior wall of the rectum.
    B   is associated with Crohn's disease.
    C   is not always solitary.
    D   is not premalignant.
    E   is associated with internal intussusception.

873. **Benign tumours of the rectum include the**
    A   keratoacanthoma.
    B   pseudopolyps.
    C   villous adenoma.
    D   endometrioma.
    E   fibroma.

874. **Villous adenomas of the rectum**
    A   must of necessity be treated by abdominoperineal excision of the rectum.
    B   tend to be small and multiple.
    C   can cause hypokalaemia.
    D   are always benign.
    E   produce mucus.

875. **Non-malignant strictures of the rectum include those that are**
   A   a spasmodic variety with fibrosis of the external sphincter due to anal fissure.
   B   postoperative after haemorrhoidectomy.
   C   due to endometriosis.
   D   due to granuloma venereum.
   E   congenital in original.

876. **Carcinoma of the rectum**
   A   is a nodule before it becomes an ulcer.
   B   is known to occur in a previously benign adenoma.
   C   spreads locally in a longitudinal manner.
   D   penetrates the fascia propria at an early stage.
   E   only exceptionally spreads downwards in lymphatics.

877. **Carcinoma of the rectum**
   A   is a squamous-celled lesion.
   B   can occur in youth.
   C   causes bleeding that is slight in amount.
   D   simulates internal haemorrhoids.
   E   is associated with juvenile polyp.

878. **In the classification of carcinoma of the rectum according to Dukes**
   A   stage A is when the growth is limited to the rectal wall.
   B   stage B is when the growth has spread to the pararectal tissues but not to nodes.
   C   stage C.1 is when secondary deposits are present in the pararectal nodes.
   D   stage C.2 means that liver metastases are present.
   E   stage D indicates that other metastases are present.

879. **Treatment of recognised value for carcinoma of the rectum includes**
   A   anterior resection.
   B   Paul Mikulicz procedure.
   C   Goodsall's ligature.
   D   abdominoperineal resection.
   E   Hartmann's operation.

880. **The anatomical features of the anal canal are manifest by**
   A   an external sphincter 2.5 cm in length.
   B   longitudinal muscle fibres mingling with those of the puborectalis.
   C   the intersphincteric plane containing parts of apocrine glands.
   D   columns of Morgagni.
   E   plum-coloured squamous epithelium.

881. **The function of the anal and pelvic floor musculature can be studied effectively by**
   A   pull-through manometry.
   B   electromyography.
   C   routine barium enema.
   D   mapping the level and angle of the anorectal ring.
   E   acupuncture.

882. **With imperforate anus**
   A   the lesion is 'low' if the bowel terminates below the pelvic floor.
   B   if 'high' can be associated with a urinary fistula.
   C   if a stenosed anus, requires a pull-through operation.
   D   if a covered anus, can be opened with scissors followed by dilatation.
   E   rectal atresia responds to dilatation.

883. **A patient with a true pilonidal sinus**
   A   has a post-anal dermoid.
   B   could well be a barber.
   C   has hair follicles in the walls of the sinus.
   D   has it within the fibres of the corrigator cutis ani.
   E   tends to get fistula in ano as a result of secondary abscesses.

884. **The reasons supporting the acquired theory of the origin of pilonidal sinus include**
   A   the occurrence of pilonidal sinus in a digital web.
   B   the age of onset.
   C   the projecting hairs having their pointed ends directed towards the opening of the sinus.
   D   hair follicles rarely being found within the walls of the sinus.
   E   association with postanal dermoids.

885. **Recognised causes of anal incontinence include**
   A   spina bifida.
   B   hyperthyroidism.
   C   pudendal nerve neuropathy.
   D   acute anal fissure.
   E   proctalgia fugax.

886. **An anal fissure is**
  A   a complication of an anal fistula.
  B   sometimes due to carcinoma of the anus.
  C   painful during defecation.
  D   a cause of acquired megacolon.
  E   due to lymphogranuloma.

887. **Internal piles**
  A   contain veins, arteries and nerves.
  B   are often symptomatic of portal hypertension.
  C   are principally three in number located at 1, 5 and 7 o'clock with the patient in the lithotomy position.
  D   are the cause of proctalgia fugax.
  E   are called second degree when they are permanently prolapsed.

888. **An acceptable solution for the injection of haemorrhoids is**
  A   5% sodium tetradecyl sulphate.
  B   5% phenol in almond or arachis oil.
  C   5% phenol in water.
  D   pure almond or arachis oil.
  E   10% dextrose solution.

889. **External haemorrhoids are simulated by**
  A   anal warts.
  B   condylomas.
  C   hypertrophic tuberculide.
  D   leucoplakia.
  E   pilonidal sinus.

890. **A thrombosed external haemorrhoid is**
  A   not unlike a semi-ripe blackcurrant in appearance.
  B   painless.
  C   a prolapsed strangulated internal haemorrhoid.
  D   a feature of Crohn's disease.
  E   best treated by injection of ethanoleate.

891. **The causes of pruritis ani include**
  A   piles.
  B   gonorrhoea.
  C   parasites.
  D   *Entamoeba histolytica*.
  E   a polypus.

892. **An ischiorectal abscess**
- A   can be tuberculous in origin.
- B   is an infective necrosis of the fat of the ischiorectal fossa.
- C   requires deroofing.
- D   should be treated entirely by antibiotics.
- E   can be followed by anal fistula.

893. **The assessment of a fistula in ano in the outpatient clinic includes**
- A   proctoscopy.
- B   probing.
- C   injection of lipiodol and x-ray.
- D   ordering an x-ray of the chest.
- E   sigmoidoscopy.

894. **Regarding fistula in ano**
- A   a high intersphincteric anal fistula runs between the internal and external sphincters along the plane of the longitudinal muscle fibres.
- B   a high intersphincteric fistula is treated by dividing the external sphincter.
- C   a high transphincteric fistula should be treated by laying the track open.
- D   a low level fistula will respond to and heal under the influence of antibiotics.
- E   a protective colostomy may be required in the treatment of a high level fistula.

895. **The causes of non-malignant strictures of the anal canal include**
- A   granuloma inguinale.
- B   Crohn's disease.
- C   endometriosis.
- D   anal chancre.
- E   yaws.

896. **Malignant tumours of the anal canal include**
- A   keratocanthoma.
- B   cylindroma.
- C   melanoma.
- D   basaloid.
- E   condylomata lata.

897. Malignant tumours of the anus

A   include basaloid tumours.
B   primarily spread to the inferior mesenteric lymph nodes.
C   are all radiosensitive.
D   simulate anal fissure.
E   are normally squamous-celled.

Chapter 18

Hernias
The umbilicus and abdominal wall

898. The boundaries of the inguinal canal include
- A anteriorly – transversalis fascia.
- B posteriorly – psoas.
- C superiorly – rectus abdominis.
- D inferiorly – inguinal ligament.
- E medially – the iliopectineal ligament (Gimbernat's).

899. The differential diagnosis of an inguinal hernia in the female includes
- A a vaginal hydrocele.
- B an encysted hydrocele of the cord.
- C a hydrocele in the canal of Nuck.
- D a femoral hernia.
- E Bartholin's cyst.

900. A strangulated inguinal hernia
- A is tense.
- B is tender.
- C has a transmitted cough impulse.
- D is irreducible.
- E requires elective surgery.

901. Regarding operation for an indirect inguinal hernia
- A it should not be performed on patients who have chronic bronchitis.
- B general anaesthesia has to be used.
- C in infants the posterior inguinal wall should be repaired.
- D in adults the internal inguinal ring usually needs to be strengthened.
- E mesh implants are mandatory.

902. A direct inguinal hernia
- A is a hernia through the transversalis fascia.
- B can extend into the scrotum.
- C can contain bladder as part of the wall of the sac.
- D has a neck which is always medial to the inferior epigastric artery.
- E is otherwise called a ventral hernia.

903. The anatomical site of the neck of a femoral hernia is the
   A   transversalis fascia.
   B   iliopectineal ligament.
   C   femoral ring.
   D   cribiform fascia.
   E   obturator foramen.

904. Clinical features characteristic of a strangulated femoral hernia include
   A   a rising pulse rate.
   B   central abdominal distension.
   C   central abdominal pain.
   D   a swelling in the groin with an expansile impulse on coughing.
   E   a varicocele.

905. Management not advised for the treatment of a femoral hernia includes
   A   Lockwood's operation.
   B   Lotheissen's operation.
   C   a truss.
   D   McEvedy's operation.
   E   Mayo's operation.

906. The complications of a femoral hernia include
   A   irreducibility.
   B   obstruction without strangulation.
   C   inflammation.
   D   Richter's hernia.
   E   hydrocele.

907. A para-umbilical hernia
   A   is a form of exomphalos.
   B   is five times more frequent in women than in men.
   C   does not strangulate.
   D   is treated by the Mayo type of operation.
   E   is associated with the appearance of intertrigo.

908. An epigastric hernia is a
   A   spigelian hernia.
   B   fatty hernia of the linea alba.
   C   type of umbilical hernia.
   D   divarication of the rectus abdominis muscles.
   E   complication of a hiatus hernia.

909. **Umbilical discharges are associated with**
   A   endometrioma.
   B   pilonidal sinus.
   C   raspberry tumour (adenoma).
   D   patent urachus.
   E   Meckel's diverticulum.

910. **Factors and conditions recognised to contribute to burst abdomen include**
   A   economy with the length of material used for abdominal closure.
   B   deep wound infection.
   C   endometrioma.
   D   jaundice.
   E   drainage through a laparotomy wound.

911. **Tearing of the inferior epigastric artery occurs**
   A   in elderly women.
   B   in muscular men.
   C   in pregnant women.
   D   at the level of the arcuate line.
   E   as a painless lump just below the umbilicus.

912. **Postoperative synergistic gangrene**
   A   is a complication of appendicitis.
   B   is a complication of drainage of an empyema thoracis.
   C   begins in the muscle layers.
   D   is a self-localising condition.
   E   requires hyperbaric oxygen therapy, if available.

913. **The desmoid tumour is**
   A   a soft fibroma.
   B   encapsulated.
   C   undergoes myxomatous degeneration.
   D   associated with Crohn's disease.
   E   contains cells like foreign body giant cells.

Chapter 19

Investigation of urinary tract
Anuria
Kidneys and ureters
The urinary bladder
The prostate and seminal vesicles
The urethra and penis
The testis and scrotum

914. **Among simple renal investigations**
  A a fixed low specific gravity of urine equates with normal renal function.
  B a dark-coloured urine is consistent with renal failure.
  C bacteriuria, if asymptomatic, excludes chronic pyelonephritis.
  D creatinine clearance is a measure of tubular function.
  E the presence of tubercle bacilli in the urine is demonstrated by means of the Papanicolaou stain.

915. **In renal imaging**
  A a plain x-ray is of little value relating to renal pathology.
  B i.v. sodium diatrizoate is allergenic.
  C retrograde ureteropyelography can be used for urothelial cytology.
  D ultrasonography gives clear imaging of the whole length of the ureters.
  E CT scanning will show invasion of the renal vein by tumour.

916. **The intravenous urogram**
  A depends upon the glomerular filtration of radio-iodine.
  B is contraindicated in patients with myelomatosis.
  C is strictly contraindicated in the presence of poor renal function.
  D can demonstrate residual urine.
  E in the early phase can produce a nephrogram.

917. **Acute renal anuria can be attributed to**
  A acute pancreatitis.
  B the crush syndrome.
  C bacteraemic shock.
  D the use of frusemide in conjunction with cephalosporins.
  E the use of intravenous dextrans.

918. **In a patient with acute renal failure**
- A   the stage of acute tubular necrosis requires fluid replacement at the rate of 1200 ml per day plus the volume of urine passed in the previous 24 hours.
- B   the stage of reversal leads rapidly to hyperkalaemia.
- C   peritoneal dialysis is effected via a fenestrated catheter inserted below the umbilicus.
- D   haemodialysis implies heparinisation.
- E   haemofiltration is a satisfactory support technique.

919. **Of the drainage procedures available for obstructive renal failure**
- A   percutaneous nephrostomy is carried out with the patient in the lateral position.
- B   the ureter can be drained by insertion of a J-stent via cystoscopy.
- C   a J-stent can be inserted via a nephrostomy.
- D   open nephrostomy need never be performed nowadays.
- E   stones in the lower ureter can be removed with the aid of a Dormia basket.

920. **With congenital abnormalities of the kidney**
- A   a urogram of horseshoe kidney shows that the lowest calyx on each side is reversed.
- B   the patients with congenital cystic kidneys tend to pass small amounts of concentrated urine.
- C   calculus can occur in cases of congenital cystic kidneys.
- D   a solitary renal cyst is not always solitary.
- E   aberrant renal vessels accentuate a hydronephrosis.

921. **Congenital cystic disease of the kidneys is**
- A   a hereditary disease transmitted by either parent.
- B   recognised to be associated with similar disease in the pancreas and lung.
- C   usually unilateral.
- D   commonly complicated by pyelonephritis.
- E   a likely indication for renal transplantation.

922. **The management of a patient with an injury to the kidney includes the use of**
- A   morphine.
- B   bed-rest.
- C   an intravenous urogram.
- D   partial nephrectomy.
- E   trimethoprim.

923. Features associated with unilateral hydronephrosis include
A incomplete urethral obstruction.
B retrocaval ureter.
C a ureterocele.
D a varicocele.
E sickle-cell disease.

924. Hydronephrosis is
A due to sudden complete obstruction to the outflow of urine from a kidney.
B characteristically a cause of haematuria.
C related to Dietl's crisis.
D associated with pregnancy.
E premalignant.

925. Urinary calculi forming in an acid urine can contain
A calcium oxalate.
B triple phosphate.
C urates.
D citrates.
E bilirubin.

926. Cystine calculi
A are likely to appear in the urinary tract of patients with cystinuria.
B are due to an inborn error of metabolism.
C contain crystals that are hexagonal.
D are radio-opaque owing to the calcium they contain.
E are soft, like beeswax.

927. Lesions known to simulate a renal calculus on x-ray include
A phleboliths.
B calcified lymph nodes.
C pure cholesterol gallstones.
D fersolate tablets.
E Tietze's disease.

928. Operative procedures employed for removal of stones from the kidney or ureter include
A nephrostomy.
B partial nephrectomy.
C extracorporeal shock-wave lithotripsy.
D push bang.
E Anderson-Hynes.

929. **Recognised associations with urinary stone formation include**
   A   paraplegia.
   B   myasthenia gravis.
   C   hypercholesteraemia.
   D   primary aldosteronism.
   E   hypoparathyroidism.

930. **A ureteric calculus**
   A   can cause strangury.
   B   is normally treated expectantly.
   C   causing colic is treated with NSAIDs.
   D   usually causes less pain than appendicitis.
   E   should be removed if the urine is infected.

931. **Clinical and pathological associations of acute pyelonephritis include**
   A   the infection being blood-borne to the kidney from a boil on the skin.
   B   *Proteus mirabilis* being the usual organism.
   C   an alkaline urine in the presence of *Escherichia coli* infection.
   D   sudden abdominal pain and vomiting.
   E   a differential diagnosis including pneumonia and acute appendicitis.

932. **In acute pyelonephritis**
   A   the infection is confined to the renal pelvis.
   B   the isotope renogram shows scattered areas of diminished uptake.
   C   there should be a search for a congenital abnormality.
   D   in the early stage the urine has many pus cells and few bacteria.
   E   treatment should not be prolonged.

933. **In chronic pyelonephritis**
   A   dull lumbar pain is present in some 60% of cases.
   B   hypertension is present in some 40% of cases.
   C   casts are frequently found in the urine.
   D   white cells in the urine may be as high as several million/ml.
   E   a presenting feature is normochromic anaemia.

934. **A pyonephrosis**
   A   is a carbuncle of the kidney.
   B   is infection of hydronephrosis.
   C   is a complication of renal calculus.
   D   can present as anaemia.
   E   can only be cured by nephrectomy.

935. Perinephric abscess is associated with
A tuberculosis.
B pyuria.
C appendix abscess.
D bacteriuria.
E scoliosis.

936. In tuberculosis of the kidney
A the patient is usually a woman aged 50 years.
B the earliest symptom is haematuria.
C the urine is acid and contains pus cells.
D changes in the pyelogram commence with loss or dysfunction of one or more calyces.
E surgical procedures are unnecessary because of advances in antituberculous chemotherapy.

937. Wilms' tumour
A is a neuroblastoma.
B arises from autonomic nerve fibres around the renal vessels.
C characteristically contains haemorrhagic areas.
D does not metastasise.
E characteristically produces erythropoietin.

938. Recognised associations with hypernephroma include
A hirsutism.
B polyuria.
C polycythaemia.
D polyposis coli.
E left inguinal hernia.

939. Regarding tumours of the kidney
A benign tumours are rare.
B a nephroblastoma is a greyish-white or pinkish-white in colour.
C a hypernephroma is a big tumour confined to the upper pole of the kidney.
D aortography shows an avascular area in the case of a tumour.
E adequate treatment depends on nephrectomy and removal of the perinephric fat.

940. The presentation of adenocarcinoma of the kidney in a woman includes
A   pyrexia.
B   polycythaemia.
C   clot colic.
D   a rapidly developing varicocele.
E   a fracture.

941. In the bladder
A   the lining epithelium is characteristically cubical.
B   detrusor fibres are generally arranged in distinct layers.
C   detrusor fibres are associated with trabeculation.
D   the internal sphincter is innervated by α-adrenergic fibres.
E   the distal urethral sphincter is composed of smooth muscle which preserves continence.

942. In complete ectopia vesicae
A   effluxes of urine from the ureteric orifices can be seen.
B   hypospadias is present.
C   a para-umbilical hernia is present.
D   the patient has a waddling gait.
E   the results of surgery are good.

943. Rupture of the bladder
A   occurs intraperitoneally in 80% of cases.
B   if intraperitoneal is characteristically caused by a fractured pelvis.
C   if extraperitoneal cannot in most cases be differentiated from rupture of the posterior urethra.
D   if intraperitoneal is an indication for lapararotomy.
E   if accidentally caused and recognised at endoscopy can be managed by a large-bored urethral catheter.

944. When the bulbous urethra is ruptured
A   retention of urine is one of the signs.
B   the patient should be encouraged to pass urine.
C   if he cannot pass urine the patient should be catheterised on the spot.
D   the urethra should be completely repaired by sutures.
E   the perineal wound, if an operation is performed, is packed not stitched.

945. In the management of acute retention of urine
A   relief by catheterisation is always necessary.
B   admission to hospital after relief is always necessary.
C   self-retainment of a catheter is by the use of the Fogarty type.
D   suprapubic puncture is contraindicated.
E   immediate prostatectomy can be performed in cases of enlarged prostate.

946. In relation to spinal shock
A   the bladder detrusor is paralysed.
B   there is overflow incontinence.
C   intermittent catheterisation is the preferred way of keeping the bladder empty.
D   where there is total sensory loss below the upper level of cord injury, recovery is unlikely.
E   eventual demonstration of intact bulbocavernous and anal reflex indicates that automatic bladder contractions may develop.

947. Recognised associations of incontinence include
A   thimble bladder.
B   spina bifida.
C   Parkinson's disease.
D   aberrant ureter in females.
E   prostatectomy.

948. Urodynamic studies in relation to incontinence have confirmed that
A   some 50% of men with BOO have detrusor instability.
B   idiopathic detrusor instability is uncommon.
C   stress incontinence is not caused by sphincter weakness.
D   chronic retention with overflow incontinence is associated with high pressures during bladder filling.
E   BOO is associated with increased voiding pressures coupled with low flow rates.

949. Procedures appropriate for types of incontinence include
A   anticholinergic drugs for small capacity bladder due to fibrosis.
B   excision of ureter and relevant part of kidney for ectopic ureter and duplex system.
C   enterocystoplasty for neurogenic dysfunction (preoperative capacity about 300 ml.).
D   artificial urinary sphincter for postprostatectomy incontinence.
E   colposuspension for true stress incontinence.

950. **In a patient with vesical calculus**
  A   nocturnal frequency is characteristic.
  B   pain is referred to the tip of the penis at the end of micturition.
  C   haematuria characteristically occurs at the beginning of micturition.
  D   there is more than a 90% chance that the stone can be demonstrated on an x-ray film.
  E   litholapaxy is a method of treatment.

951. **Oxalate calculi**
  A   grow rapidly.
  B   have a smooth, rounded surface.
  C   are primarily white in colour.
  D   form in an alkaline urine.
  E   are radiolucent.

952. **Strangury is the term applied to**
  A   painful piles.
  B   a tight feeling in the neck.
  C   urinary frequency.
  D   passage of a few drops of urine, often blood-stained, after painful straining.
  E   faecal impaction.

953. **Diverticulum of the bladder**
  A   is usually congenital in origin.
  B   is lined by bladder mucosa.
  C   can be symptomless.
  D   is not always obvious on cystoscopy.
  E   can be demonstrated by ultrasound.

954. **Recognised associations with urinary fistula include**
  A   Crohn's disease.
  B   pyonephrosis.
  C   anterior colporrhaphy.
  D   Hunner's ulcer.
  E   imperforate anus.

955. **Low urinary tract infection**
  A   can be secondary to renal tuberculosis.
  B   is associated with oestrogen deficiency.
  C   does not commonly cause haematuria.
  D   is more common in men than in women.
  E   is treated with trimethoprim as a front line drug.

956. **Hunner's ulcer**
    A   is a male complaint.
    B   is characteristically a linear bleeding ulcer.
    C   results in a flaccid bladder.
    D   is associated with lymphocytic infiltration.
    E   is premalignant.

957. **In bilharziasis of the bladder**
    A   *Schistosoma haematobium* enters the circulation after being swallowed.
    B   the male worm is longer than the female worm.
    C   urticaria is an early clinical feature.
    D   a squamous-celled carcinoma commences as a papilloma.
    E   metronidazole therapy effects a cure.

958. **Betanaphthylamine, bilharzia and magenta are related in terms of**
    A   carcinoma of the colon.
    B   carcinoma of the cervix.
    C   bronchial tumours.
    D   bladder tumours.
    E   carcinoma of the stomach.

959. **There is a recognised association between**
    A   viruses and warts.
    B   warts and papillomas.
    C   bladder papillomas and bladder carcinoma.
    D   bladder carcinoma and carcinoma of the prostate.
    E   carcinoma of the prostate and osteosclerotic metastases.

960. **Clinical features characteristic of papilloma of the bladder include**
    A   clot retention.
    B   painless haematuria.
    C   periodic haematuria.
    D   pain in the perineum.
    E   rigor.

961. **Characteristic features of malignant villous tumour of the bladder are that**
    A   the villi are elongated like a sea anemone.
    B   the growth tends to be predunculated.
    C   the growth may ulcerate.
    D   the growth may become encrusted with urinary salts.
    E   if two tumours are present it is a sure sign of malignancy.

962. In the diagnosis and management of malignant bladder tumours
- **A** intermittent haematuria is significant.
- **B** an intravenous urogram is the mainstay of diagnosis.
- **C** assessment includes the use of the TNM classification.
- **D** a small biopsy settles the diagnosis.
- **E** the tumours are radio-insensitive.

963. There is a recognised association between hyperchloraemic acidosis and
- **A** urethrostomy.
- **B** potassium depletion.
- **C** osteomalacia.
- **D** ureterosigmoidostomy.
- **E** pyelostomy.

964. Benign prostatic hypertrophy
- **A** affects the submucosal group of glands.
- **B** includes enlargement of the prostatic glands proper of the outer peripheral zone.
- **C** can cause prostatism without bladder outflow obstruction (BOO).
- **D** can depress erythropoietin.
- **E** is related to increased oestrogenic effects.

965. Bladder outflow obstruction is characteristically associated with
- **A** postmicturition dribbling.
- **B** bladder neck hypertrophy.
- **C** residual urine.
- **D** pain.
- **E** enuresis.

966. The management of benign prostatic hypertrophy (BPH) includes
- **A** prostatectomy for frequency.
- **B** blood transfusion.
- **C** T.U.R.P.
- **D** prostatic stents.
- **E** bladder neck incision.

967. The complications of prostatectomy operations include
- **A** water intoxication.
- **B** bacteriaemia.
- **C** bladder neck contracture.
- **D** retrograde ejaculation.
- **E** urethral stricture.

968. **Bladder outflow obstruction (BOO) caused by the bladder neck**
A is characteristically associated with Peyronie's disease.
B can affect women and children as well as men.
C is associated with muscle hypertrophy of the internal sphincter.
D can result in a vesical diverticulum.
E is best treated by transurethral incision of the bladder neck.

969. **The natural history of carcinoma of the prostate includes the fact that**
A about 20% of cases of prostatic obstruction prove to be due to carcinoma.
B tiny neoplasms found in serial sections of the prostate in 15% of men aged over 50 are examples of dormant cancer.
C the growth spreads early through the fascia of Denonvilliers.
D bony metastases tend to be osteosclerotic.
E lymph nodes do become involved.

970. **Of the treatments for carcinoma of the prostate**
A radical prostatectomy is suitable for T3/T4 (TNM) tumours.
B radical radiotherapy is applicable for T1/T2 tumours.
C general radiotherapy is unhelpful.
D a T.U.R.P. is applicable if there is associated BOO.
E aminoglutethimide is applicable in advanced cases as it inhibits androgens.

971. **Features indicative of a diagnosis of chronic prostatitis include**
A referred pain down the legs.
B infected seminal vesicles.
C in the three glass test, prostatitis is present if threads are seen in the last glass.
D haematuria obtained by a catheter specimen of urine.
E an enlarged oedematous verumontanum revealed by urethroscopy.

972. **Extravasation of urine in cases of complete rupture of the bulbous urethra for anatomical reasons**
A cannot pass behind the midperineal point.
B can pass into the inguinal canals.
C can pass into the upper half of the thigh.
D cannot pass up the abdominal wall beneath the deep layer of the superficial fascia.
E can pass into the scrotum.

973. **Urethral meatal ulcer in male children is associated with**
   A   circumcision.
   B   ammoniacal dermatitis.
   C   passing blood.
   D   Reiter's disease.
   E   pinhole meatus.

974. **Gonorrhoea**
   A   is due to a gram-positive diplococcus.
   B   can cause acute suppurative arthritis.
   C   can occur in the anus and rectum.
   D   begins by penetration by the gonococcus of the epithelium of the glans penis.
   E   characteristically presents as acute retention of urine.

975. **In Reiter's disease**
   A   conjunctivitis occurs.
   B   acute hydrarthrosis is present.
   C   a urethral smear reveals streptococci.
   D   keratoderma blenorrhagicum of the heel is a concurrent manifestation.
   E   a urethral smear reveals gonococci.

976. **Symptoms of urethral stricture include**
   A   morning 'dewdrop'.
   B   dribbling urine after micturition.
   C   gleet.
   D   hesitancy.
   E   hydrocele.

977. **The complications of urethral stricture include**
   A   Dupuytren's contracture.
   B   hydronephrosis.
   C   periurethral abscess.
   D   hernia.
   E   Peyronie's disease.

978. **Gonorrhoea in the female is related to**
   A   Bartholinitis.
   B   vulval warts.
   C   ophthalmia neonatorum.
   D   ureterocele.
   E   Reiter's disease.

979. **Regarding balanoposthitis**
  A   inflammation of the prepuce is called posthitis.
  B   inflammation of the glans is called balanitis.
  C   a cancer may be the cause of balanoposthitis.
  D   a chancre is not a cause of balanoposthitis.
  E   operation is unnecessary.

980. **Concerning lymphogranuloma venereum**
  A   the Frei test should be positive.
  B   it is due to *Donovania granulomatis*.
  C   the primary lesion is a vesicle surrounded by erythema that is a bright beefy red.
  D   it is a cause of rectal stricture.
  E   it responds to suphonamides.

981. **Granuloma inguinale is**
  A   synonymous with lymphogranuloma venerum.
  B   caused by a virus.
  C   manifest by an ulcer in the groin.
  D   complicated by Peyronie's disease.
  E   treatable by oxytetracycline.

982. **Condylomata acuminata**
  A   are not sexually transmitted.
  B   are associated with psoriasis.
  C   are caused by chlamydia infection.
  D   are caused by varieties of human papilloma virus.
  E   occur only in men.

983. **Precancerous lesions of the penis include**
  A   leucoplakia of the glans.
  B   Littritis.
  C   chronic penile papilloma.
  D   Paget's disease (erythroplasia).
  E   paraphimosis.

984. Regarding carcinoma of the penis

A circumcision in childhood gives complete immunity against the condition.

B it is a disease of the elderly.

C enlargement of the inguinal lymph nodes means that metastasis has taken place.

D radiotherapy gives good results with small well-differentiated tumours.

E total amputation of the penis means that the patient will have a perineal urethrostomy.

985. There is a recognised clinical association between

A Reiter's disease and urethritis.

B phimosis and carcinoma of the penis.

C ectopia vesicae and pubic bone deficiency.

D catheters and urethral stricture.

E spermatocele and enlarged prostate.

986. Incomplete descent of the testis

A is arrest of the testis in some part of its path to the scrotum.

B occurs in 30% of premature infants.

C does not affect the internal secretory activity of the testis.

D is commonest on the left side.

E is present if the testis on traction cannot be made to touch the bottom of the scrotum.

987. Torsion of the testis is

A common.

B related to anomalies in the anchorage of the testis.

C difficult to distinguish from a strangulated inguinal hernia.

D unknown before puberty.

E treated by bed-rest and cold compresses.

988. Recognised associations with a varicocele include

A the right side of the body.

B varicose veins.

C wearing tight pants.

D oligospermia.

E hydronephrosis.

989. A hydrocele
A   is not translucent.
B   contains fluid that clots spontaneously.
C   can communicate with the peritoneal cavity.
D   is separate from the testis.
E   can obscure a hernia.

990. Regarding the treatment of a hydrocele
A   the fluid is removed with a Trucut needle.
B   tapping nearly always results in a cure.
C   a haematocele may follow tapping.
D   Lord's operation of ruffing the tunica at the edge of the testis is a suitable procedure.
E   orchiectomy is preferable.

991. Clinical associations with hydrocele of the cord include
A   exomphalos.
B   absent testis.
C   hydatid disease.
D   lateral mobility.
E   lack of translucency.

992. The complications of a primary hydrocele include
A   rupture.
B   calcification.
C   a spermatocele.
D   a chylocele.
E   herniation.

993. Cysts of the epididymis
A   contain barley water-like fluid.
B   are spermatoceles.
C   are tense cysts.
D   are situated in front of the body of the testis.
E   transilluminate like a chinese lantern.

994. In the management of what one thinks is acute epididymo-orchitis one must be aware that
A   the swelling may really be neoplastic.
B   the scrotal skin may become adherent and the epididymis may discharge.
C   the swelling may be due to tuberculosis.
D   bed-rest is unnecessary.
E   the urine should be made acid.

995. **Clinical features of tuberculous epididymitis include**
  A involvement of the globus major.
  B firm and craggy nature.
  C a thickened 'beaded' vas.
  D early involvement of the testis.
  E the semen yielding tubercle bacilli on culture.

996. **Regarding neoplasms of the testis**
  A a seminoma arises in the interstitial cells of the testis.
  B a teratoma arises from the mediastinum testis.
  C a Leydig-cell tumour arises from the rete testis.
  D the peak incidence of teratoma testis is between 20–25 years of age.
  E macroscopically the seminoma is homogeneous, pink or cream in colour.

997. **The clinical presentation of a seminoma of the testis includes**
  A an upper abdominal mass.
  B hirsutism.
  C a left supraclavicular swelling.
  D osteosclerotic metastases.
  E a painful swelling in the scrotum.

998. **The action to be taken when a clinical diagnosis of neoplasm of the testis is made includes**
  A a chest x-ray.
  B orchiectomy (or exploration).
  C dissection of inguinal lymph nodes.
  D vasectomy on the contralateral side.
  E radiotherapy.

999. **Concerning the management and prognosis of malignant tumours of the testis**
  A only 25% with seminoma without metastases survive five years if treated by orchiectomy and radiotherapy.
  B 80% with teratoma (differentiated) without metastases survive five years if treated by orchiectomy and radiotherapy.
  C seminomas are highly radio-insensitive.
  D radiotherapy can be given by a cobalt or linear accelerator x-ray unit.
  E an x-ray of the chest and an IVP are essential in assessment before radiotherapy is given.

1000. **Elephantiasis of the scrotum is associated with**

    A   lymphogranuloma venereum.

    B   *Wucheria Bancroftii* infection.

    C   sebaceous cysts.

    D   Fournier's gangrene.

    E   the 'Elephant man'.

1001. **Primary carcinoma of the scrotum**

    A   is almost unknown in Asiatic countries.

    B   spreads to inguinal and external iliac lymph nodes.

    C   is columnar-celled.

    D   is a recognised complication of elephantiasis.

    E   has an association with the kangri.

Part Two

Answers ('true' completions)

Chapter 1

1. A E
2. C D E
3. A B
4. A B D
5. A B C
6. D E
7. A B C D
8. B
9. E
10. A B C E
11. B
12. B C D
13. B
14. C D
15. C
16. A B D
17. C
18. C D E
19. A B
20. D
21. A B C
22. A B C
23. B D E
24. A B C E
25. C D E
26. B D E
27. A B E
28. B
29. D
30. D
31. A B C D
32. C D E
33. D
34. C D E
35. C D E
36. A B C
37. B C E
38. A B C E
39. A B C
40. A B C
41. A B C E

42. A D
43. B D E
44. A B C D
45. A B C D
46. A C D
47. A B C
48. A C D E
49. C D E
50. NONE
51. C
52. B
53. A B C D E
54. A B E
55. C
56. B
57. C
58. A
59. E
60. A
61. A D E
62. B D
63. A B C D
64. B D E
65. A B D
66. B
67. A C D E

Chapter 2

68. A B C D E
69. A E
70. A C D
71. A E
72. A D
73. A B E
74. A D E
75. A C E
76. A B D
77. A C D E
78. C E
79. A B E
80. D
81. C
82. B C
83. A C D
84. A B
85. D E
86. A D E
87. C E
88. NONE
89. C
90. B C E
91. A C D
92. C D
93. C E
94. A B C
95. D E
96. A B C D
97. A C E
98. A D E
99. A B C D E
100. A B C E
101. C D E
102. C D E
103. A B C
104. A B D
105. A D E
106. B C D
107. A D E
108. B C E

109. A B C
110. A B C
111. A B C D E
112. C E
113. C D
114. A B E

Chapter 3

115. B
116. A B C
117. A B C
118. C D E
119. C
120. A E
121. B
122. A B C
123. B D E
124. A B D E
125. B C
126. A B E
127. A B E
128. A B D E
129. B C
130. A C D
131. C
132. D E
133. B D
134. C
135. C
136. D
137. D
138. A B C
139. D
140. E
141. A B C D
142. C E
143. A C D
144. E
145 A C
146. C D
147. A D
148. A B C D E
149. A B D
150. A B C D E
151. A B C D E
152. C D E

Chapter 4

153. D	194. A B D
154. C	195. C D
155. C	196. C
156. E	197. A C E
157. A B D	198. B C D
158. C	199. B C D
159. B	200. B
160. C E	201. C
161. C	202. A B C
162. A D E	203. B
163. C	204. D
164. B E	205. A B C E
165. NONE	206. A B C D
166. C	207. B C D E
167. A C E	208. C
168. A B C D E	209. C E
169. A B D	210. A B D
170. D E	211. B
171. A B E	212. B
172. A B C D E	213. C D
173. A B	214. B E
174. B	215. B C
175. D	216. A B
176. B C D	217. A B C
177. A B C	218. C D E
178. C	
179. E	
180. D	
181. C D	
182. B D E	
183. A D E	
184. E	
185. A B D	
186. B	
187. D	
188. B C E	
189. B	
190. E	
191. B C D E	
192. A B D E	
193. B D E	

Chapter 5

Chapter 6

280. A C E	321. B C D
281. A B	322. B C D
282. D E	323. C
283. B C D	324. B D
284. A B C D	325. A B C D
285. NONE	326. A B D
286. A B E	327. C
287. B D E	328. A C D
288. B C	329. B D
289. C	330. D
290. A D	331. D E
291. A B C	332. A B D
292. A C D	333. B D E
293. A C	334. B C D E
294. A D E	335. A B D E
295. C	336. A B C
296. C	
297. B E	
298. A C E	
299. B E	
300. A B E	
301. A C D E	
302. A B D E	
303. B C D	
304. A C D E	
305. B C D	
306. B C	
307. A B C D	
308. A C E	
309. A B D	
310. B C E	
311. C D E	
312. A D E	
313. A B E	
314. C D E	
315. C	
316. A B C	
317. B D E	
318. B C	
319. B C	
320. B D E	

Chapter 7

337. B C D
338. A B E
339. A B C D E
340. C
341. A B D
342. A B D
343. C
344. C
345. B C
346. A B C D E
347. E
348. C
349. A B C D E
350. B C D
351. A B D
352. B D E
353. A C D
354. A E
355. A B C E
356. D
357. A
358. A B C D E
359. B
360. C D E
361. E
362. C E
363. A B C D
364. C D E
365. A D E
366. B C D E
367. C
368. B E
369. A B D
370. C
371. A B C

Chapter 8

372. A C D E
373. B D
374. A D E
375. B E
376. A B C D E
377. C D E
378. B D
379. A B C D
380. C D
381. C D E
382. C D
383. A B D
384. B D
385. A B C E
386. A B C D E
387. B E
388. A B D
389. A B D
390. A B D E
391. B C D E
392. C D E
393. C E
394. A B E
395. A B E
396. B C E
397. B D E
398. B C
399. A D
400. C E
401. A B E
402. B C D E
403. E
404. C
405. A B D E
406. A C D
407. A C
408. A C D E
409. B E
410. C
411. E
412. D E

413. A B D
414. D E
415. A B C
416. A D
417. B C D E
418. B C D
419. B E
420. C E
421. A B C D E
422. A B E
423. D E
424. B C
425. A
426. C D
427. C
428. A D
429. A D E
430. C D E
431. B C D
432. A B C D
433. C E
434. B C D E
435. A B C E
436. A C E
437. A B C D E
438. A C D E
439. B D E
440. A B C D E
441. C D E
442. A B C D
443. A C E
444. A B C E
445. A B C
446. A B C E
447. B C D

Chapter 9

448. A B
449. B C E
450. D
451. A B E
452. A B D
453. A C D
454. A D E
455. D
456. B
457. A B E
458. B C D
459. B C E
460. B E
461. C D
462. C
463. B C
464. A B C
465. D
466. A B C
467. A B C
468. A
469. B
470. A C D E
471. B C D E
472. A B C
473. A B D
474. D
475. B C D
476. E
477. A B C D
478. B D
479. B E
480. A B C E
481. A B C D E
482. A B C E
483. B D
484. A C D
485. A B C
486. A C D E
487. B C E
488. B C

489. B D E
490. D
491. A D E
492. A B D E
493. A C D E
494. A D E
495. A B C D E
496. C D E
497. A B C
498. B C D E
499. A D E
500. A B C E
501. C
502. A B C E
503. D
504. A C E
505. E
506. A B D E
507. A C
508. B C
509. A B E
510. C D
511. B
512. E
513. D
514. NONE
515. A B C
516. A B C
517. A D
518. B
519. C D E
520. B D
521. A
522. C
523. A B E
524. C D E

Chapter 10

525. A D E
526. A
527. C D
528. A B C
529. A B C D E
530. A B D
531. A B C E
532. C D E
533. A
534. A B C D
535. B C D
536. D
537. A B D
538. B D
539. B D
540. A B D
541. A B
542. A D
543. A C E
544. D
545. B
546. A D E
547. C D
548. C D E
549. A C D E
550. C D E
551. E
552. A D
553. B
554. A B D

Chapter 11

555. D E
556. D E
557. B
558. B
559. C E
560. A C E
561. C D
562. D E
563. A B E
564. B C D E
565. B C E
566. E
567. A C
568. A B C D
569. A B E
570. A B E
571. B C D E
572. A B E
573. A D
574. B E
575. A B D
576. B D
577. A B C
578. A C D
579. A B C
580. A B C
581. A B C D E
582. A B
583. A B D
584. D E
585. C D
586. B C D
587. A B C D
588. A C E
589. A C D
590. A C D
591. D E
592. A B
593. A B C D
594. A B D
595. C D E

596. A D E
597. A B C D
598. B E
599. B E
600. A B C
601. A C D E
602. A B D E
603. C D E

Chapter 12

604. A B D E
605. A C
606. C E
607. D E
608. C
609. B E
610. A D E
611. B C
612. C D E
613. A B D
614. A
615. B C D
616. C D
617. B C D
618. A B C
619. A D E
620. A B C E
621. A B
622. A C
623. B C
624. A
625. A E
626. A E
627. B
628. A B C
629. A E
630. A B C D
631. A E
632. A B C D
633. B

Chapter 13

634. A B C
635. A B C D
636. A B D
637. A C D
638. C D E
639. A B C
640. A B C E
641. A B E
642. D E
643. A D
644. A B C
645. C D
646. A B C E
647. A B C D
648. B C E
649. A B D
650. A B D E
651. C D
652. A C D
653. C D E
654. B C D
655. A B C
656. A
657. B D
658. A B E
659. A B C D E
660. B C E
661. E
662. B C E
663. A B E
664. A C
665. A B C
666. B C D
667. A B C D
668. A B C E
669. A D
670. A B D
671. A C D
672. B C D E
673. A B D E
674. C D

675. A B D E
676. A B C E
677. A B C D E
678. B D
679. B D E
680. A B E
681. A B C
682. A B C E

Chapter 14

683. C E
684. A B C
685. A C D
686. B C E
687. A B C E
688. C D
689. B C E
690. A E
691. NONE
692. D
693. A B C D E
694. B D E
695. B C D E
696. B D
697. A B C
698. B C
699. B C E
700. A C D E
701. A B D E
702. A C
703. A B C D
704. A B D
705. A B C
706. D E
707. B
708. C D
709. C D
710. A C D
711. B D E
712. C D E
713. D E
714. A B C E
715. B C D E
716. E
717. A B C D E
718. A B C E
719. D E
720. NONE
721. B C
722. B C D
723. A B D

724. B
725. A B
726. C D
727. B E
728. A B D E
729. A B C
730. B C E
731. B C D
732. C D
733. D
734. A D
735. D
736. A
737. A B C E
738. B E
739. A C D
740. B

Chapter 15

741. B C E
742. B D E
743. A B E
744. A B E
745. C E
746. A B C
747. B C D
748. A C
749. A
750. A B E
751. A B
752. B D E
753. B C E
754. B C D E
755. A
756. A C E
757. A E
758. A E
759. A D E
760. B C D
761. B C E
762. A D E
763. B C E
764. A B C
765. B C D
766. A E
767. A C E
768. A B C
769. C D E
770. B D E
771. A D
772. A B C E
773. C D
774. B E
775. A D
776. A B C
777. NONE
778. A B C D E
779. A B D E
780. A B C E
781. B C D E

782. A E
783. B C D E
784. A B C D
785. C E
786. B C E
787. C E
788. B C E
789. B C D E
790. A E
791. A B C
792. A B C E
793. C D E
794. B C D
795. B
796. E
797. A B D E
798. B C D E
799. A B C D
800. A B C
801. A D E
802. A
803. B C D
804. A B E
805. D E
806. B C E
807. A B C
808. A D E
809. C E
810. A B C
811. A B C
812. B D
813. A C E

Chapter 16

814. A B C
815. B C D
816. E
817. A D
818. A C D E
819. A B
820. B C D
821. A B C E
822. A B C E
823. A C D
824. A
825. B D
826. C D
827. A B C D
828. A B C
829. A C D
830. B C D
831. A D E
832. A D E
833. C
834. C
835. A C
836. A B C
837. B C E
838. A B C
839. A B D E
840. C E
841. A B C D E
842. A B
843. A E
844. A D E
845. A B D
846. C D E
847. E
848. B C E
849. B C D
850. B C D
851. B C D
852. A B
853. A B D E
854. B

855. NONE
856. A B C
857. C D E
858. B D
859. B C D
860. A B C D E
861. B
862. A B C D
863. A C
864. C D

Chapter 17

865. D E
866. B
867. B C
868. A C D
869. A B C E
870. B C D
871. B C D
872. B C D E
873. B C D E
874. C E
875. A B C E
876. A B E
877. B C D E
878. A B C E
879. A D E
880. B C D
881. A B D
882. A B D
883. B
884. A B D
885. A C
886. B C D
887. A
888. B
889. A B D
890. A
891. A B C D E
892. A B C E
893. A D E
894. A E
895. B C
896. C D
897. A D E

Chapter 18

898. D
899. C D
900. A B C D
901. D
902. A B C D
903. A
904. A B C
905. C E
906. A B C D
907. B D E
908. B
909. A B C D E
910. A B D E
911. A B C D
912. A B E
913. C E

Chapter 19

914. B
915. B C E
916. B D E
917. A B C D
918. C D E
919. B C E
920. A C D E
921. A B D E
922. A B C D E
923. B C E
924. C D
925. A C
926. A B C E
927. A B D
928. A B C D
929. A
930. B C E
931. A D E
932. B C
933. A B D E
934. B C D
935. A C E
936. C D
937. A
938. C
939. A B E
940. A B C E
941. C D
942. A C D
943. C D E
944. A E
945. B E
946. A B C D E
947. A B C D E
948. A D E
949. B C D E
950. B D E
951. C
952. D
953. B C D E
954. A B C E

955. A B E
956. B D
957. C
958. D
959. A B C E
960. A B C
961. A B C D E
962. A C
963. B C D
964. A C D E
965. B C E
966. B C D E
967. A B D E
968. B C D E
969. A D E
970. B D E
971. A B E
972. A E
973. A B C E
974. B C
975. A B D
976. A B C
977. B C D
978. A B C
979. A B C
980. A D E
981. C E
982. D
983. A C D
984. D E
985. A B C D
986. A B E
987. B C
988. B C D
989. C E
990. C D
991. D
992. A B E
993. C E
994. A B C
995. A B C E

996. D E
997. A C E
998. A B E
999. D E
1000. A B
1001. A B

NOTES

NOTES

NOTES

NOTES

NOTES

NOTES

NOTES

NOTES

NOTES

NOTES